RISING STRONGER SERIES™:

Loving and Essential Paths to Healing After Losing a Child™

Authors:

Dr. Pauline E. Wallner, D.M., et. al.

DR. PAULINE E. WALLNER, D.M., et. al.

RISING STRONGER SERIES™:

Loving and Essential Paths to Healing After Losing a Child™

Author:

Dr. Pauline E. Wallner, D.M., et. al.

Contributing Authors:

- Ms. Annette M. Nalty, B.Sc. Finance, MBA
- Ms. Valdete A. Paiva-Cargill (Mimi), Chef
- Ms. Beth M. Wilson-Smalling, BA
- Ms. Valerie M. Shelton
- Ms. Hyacinth Williams-Blake, RN, MSN, CCRN
- Ms. Ingrid (Anonymous)
- Ms. Sharon A. White-Answer-Carter, CNA

Published By

NMWB Global Management Services, LLC
www.paulinewallnerspeaks.com www.nmwbglobal.com

RISING STRONGER SERIES™:

Loving and Essential Paths to Healing After Losing a Child™

Author:

Dr. Pauline E. Wallner, D.M., et. al.

Contributing Authors:

Ms. Annette M. Nalty, B.Sc. Finance, MBA
Ms. Valdete A. Paiva-Cargill (Mimi), Chef
Ms. Beth M. Wilson-Smalling, BA
Ms. Valerie M. Shelton
Ms. Hyacinth Williams-Blake, RN, MSN, CCRN
Ms. Ingrid (Anonymous)
Ms. Sharon A. White-Answer-Carter, CNA

Foreword

Dr. Michael B. Grossman, DM, MSN, RN

TABLE OF CONTENTS

ABOUT THE AUTHOR

Dr. Pauline Elizabeth Wallner (nee, Nooks) is the managing director of NMWB Global Management Services, LLC. As an author, speaker, coach, and workshop trainer/facilitator, she brings the audience alive with innovative, artistic, and vivid presentations of organizational and behavioral challenges to stimulate solutions-oriented environments. She has first-hand knowledge of global cultures and competencies, having lived, worked, taught, traveled, or facilitated seminars worldwide. As an action-learning consultant, Dr. Wallner travels worldwide with mid-level and executive teams from diverse corporations, coaching them to seek solutions to real-world problems and close performance gaps.

Dr. Wallner created the Rising Stronger Series™ to encourage families, friends, clients, and readers to adopt a healthier mindset to alleviate pain, worry, fear, and anxiety. She inspires both contributors and readers to navigate life's impediments by creating balance in four key areas: emotional, physical, mental, and spiritual.

ABOUT THE CONTRIBUTING AUTHORS

Annette M. Nalty, B.Sc. Finance, MBA

Ms. Annette P. Nalty, B.Sc. Finance, MBA migrated from Kingston, Jamaica, over thirty years ago. As a United States Airforce spouse, she has lived in several states as well as Germany. Having traveled throughout Europe, Middle East, Asia, and the Caribbean, she is an inclusive leader, an enthusiastic volunteer with several organizations, and an advocate for the unrepresented. Throughout her corporate tenure, she has worked in several industries as a data center analyst, senior accountant and financial analyst, and corporate controller.

Valdete A. Paiva–Cargill (Mimi), Chef

Ms. Valdete A. Paiva–Cargill (Mimi), as family and friends fondly know her, is a native of Brazil. She has lived in the United States for several decades and is an accomplished Chef. Val is known for her irresistible cuisine, vibrant personality, and warm hospitality. She is both a humanitarian and voracious comedian at heart. Her knack for contagious self–deprecating humor allows her audience to see the brighter side of tragedies. Currently, Ms. Cargill is completing a bachelor's degree at the University of Maine at Augusta.

Beth M. Wilson–Smalling, B.A. Business Management

As a Jamaican migrant, Ms. Beth M. Wilson–Smalling has lived in the United States for more than thirty years. Beth's career accomplishments include computer programming in the banking and financial management industries. As the current CEO of Swags 'N' Stuff, LLC, interior design and *window* covering experts, she provides blinds, shades, and drapery for residential and commercial clients. Additionally, her clientele includes the expansive movie industry and interior architects with whom she has demonstrated distinguished proficiencies.

Valerie M. Shelton

For several years before her debut in the United States of America, Ms. Valerie M. Shelton joined the banking industry after leaving high school. She worked in several management positions, leaving as Personnel Manager. She worked with Broward County Housing Authority for twenty-three years before retiring as Property Manager a few years ago. Known for her approachable and introverted demeanor, Ms. Shelton, widely respected for her assertive leadership style, values faith, family, friends, fellowship, and community.

Hyacinth Blake, RN, MSN, CCRN

Ms. Hyacinth Blake, RN, MSN, CCRN, migrated to Florida in the early 1980s and has lived there ever since. She has been in the healthcare industry for several decades and is considered an expert in her field. As an advocate for continuing education, she mentors and coaches junior staff members to embrace higher learning. Ms. Blake inspires, sponsors, and supports various community initiatives. She savors time spent traveling with her daughter and family.

Ingrid (Anonymous)

Ms. Ingrid Anonymous has lived in the United States of America for over twenty years. She worked with a computer technology trailblazing entity and as a respected consumer products manager for several years. As a pillar of her community, she is currently retired and spends valuable time traveling with her children and grandchildren. As an anonymous contributor to this book, she hopes no one else will experience the pain she has had to endure. Her objective is to help readers alleviate the anguish that grief brings in healthier settings.

Sharon A. White-Answer-Carter, CNA

Ms. Sharon A. White-Answer-Carter attended Edna Manley School of Performing Arts in Kingston, Jamaica. She migrated to the United States fifteen years ago and currently lives in Boston, Massachusetts. As a well-respected Certified Nursing Assistant (CNA) attending to seniors' needs in Massachusetts, she has a big personality; loves to entertain, travel, and host her grandchildren. She is a connoisseur of fashion designing, baking, and culinary arts. She is a well-esteemed Mistress of Ceremonies.

RISING STRONGER SERIES™

DEDICATION

We dedicate this book to the memories of the children gone too soon and not forgotten:

Cleveland George Nooks
Corey O'Neil Nalty
Melanie K. Cargill-Barbour
Christopher Craig Anthony Taylor
Wayne Vincent Shelton
Renee Misha-Gaye Williams
Dennis & Zach (Anonymous)
Georgia A. Green-Lee

"Even as we mourn our loss and celebrate the lives of our dearly departed children, we will never forget to live for our spouse, children, family, friends, and communities."

"Do your best to use the storms as anchors for the future. Only you truly know what you are feeling today. Your thoughts can spiral out of control if you let them. Phone a friend. Call a sponsor. Call a hotline. Don't let anyone tell you that positive thinking alone will solve every problem you are having. When your sadness or depression is about to cause you to walk out of a job or make unhealthy choices, a "gear shift" is necessary. Put healthy actions to your thoughts."
Pauline E. Wallner (nee, Nooks)

FOREWORD

They say there's nothing worse than losing a child. As a pediatric nurse for over 40 years, I have seen my fair share of families lose a child. Indeed, it is always devastating. The usual rationalizations like *"He led a good life," "He fulfilled all his dreams,"* and *"He left the lasting legacy"* just do not work. However, the one consolation is your ability to choose how to interpret what has happened. That is what Victor Frankl, an Austrian psychiatrist who survived the Holocaust, said in his book *Man's Search for Meaning.* Frankl survived through his will to remain stronger than those who tried to oppress him. All of this is logical, intellectual thinking. They say, *"in the battle between emotion and intellect, emotion always wins."* Losing a child is a devastating emotional event. We believe the *normal* process of life is for children to outlive their parents, yet the statistics show that 2% of parents will lose a child. For those parents who do lose a child, the statistics do not change the situation. It is prevalent for parents who have lost a child to say, *"I think about my child every day,"* and while those thoughts are painful, would you want to erase their memory?

There are constant reminders every time you attend an event and think, *"my child never experienced this."*

Unfortunately, *"tragedy happens, and life goes on."* How you handle those challenges is what matters.

I was honored by Dr. Wallner's request to write the second book's foreword in the Rising Stronger Series™. I am very inspired by her stories of always rising stronger. Despite many challenges, Pauline always finds sensible ways to rise stronger, which is an inspiration for all of us. It is a famous view that the most significant breakthroughs in life come on the heels of some suffering. While I would not suggest that people lose a child on purpose, many people leave the experience stronger.

I always say it is a gift as a nurse to be invited into people's lives at their most vulnerable moments. I have flashes of every loss I have experienced each time a patient or family member asks me, *"why is this happening?"* I do not have a magical answer that can provide them comfort. I can appreciate that my presence in those dark moments may be enough.

Several years ago, my cousin called me and said that a good friend had been given a terrible terminal prognosis for her five-year-old child. Can you imagine a physician telling you your child has only six months to live? My cousin asked me if I would talk to the mother, which I agreed to do. Based on my extensive experience, I told her I would not recommend spending the six months chasing after a miracle cure. I told her, *"I realize that your instinct as a mother is to do the best to save your child's life."* However, *"I suggest you make your child as comfortable as possible in her final months."* Much to my surprise, the family listened to me. I see them every couple of years, and they always thank me for the sage advice.

My wisdom comes on the heels of watching many families destroyed after the loss of a young one. This situation is the reality for parents who put their child through unnecessary procedures and treatments that did not significantly impact the outcome. Most of those parents said, *"if I knew this was going to happen, I would not have put my child through all of it."* Unfortunately, very few physicians have the guts to say, *"There's nothing I can do to change the outcome substantively."* Rabbi Harold Kushner wrote a famous book called *"Why Do Bad Things Happen to Good People?"* He suggested it was not worth asking why because we will never have an answer as to why. The problem is not just losing a child to illness. My daughter lost her best friend in a plane crash at her school. She was only six years old.

Why did my daughter survive and her best friend die? I am not sure there is an answer to that question, but our emotional mind wants to know why the loss happened. There are also situations of loss like accidents, murder, suicide, kidnappings, runaways, or a child that just does not want to talk to a parent anymore. Regardless of the cause, the emotional trauma for the parent is the same. My mother-in-law lost a 52-year-old son to cancer. She said it was more difficult than losing a younger child, as she had 52 years to love and adore him, so the loss was even more significant. It is not a competition over who has got the "greatest worst" story. Loss is a loss, and everyone grieves in their way.

I used to wonder why people suffer. When you see a child dying, watch a parent lose a child, or watch any loved one lose somebody, it is easy to wonder why we need to suffer. When I lost my brother three months after my brother-in-law had died, the answer came to me. I realized we could not watch him suffer any further. When a person is in a persistent vegetative coma, it is possible to sit there, care, and hope for a miracle. Yet, when you see someone suffering in pain, it is hard to justify that and more comfortable to say, *"I can't watch this anymore. Let him die in peace."* Some people say letting someone die is *playing God*. Keeping someone alive with machines, medications, and treatments that will not substantively change the situation, is *playing God.*

Ram Dass was a psychologist and spiritual leader who spent a major part of his career working in hospice and said the most important way to support someone who is grieving is to be present. He wrote the following later to the parents of a young child who died:

> *"Dear Steve and Anita*
>
> *Rachel finished her work on earth and left the stage in a manner that leaves those of us left behind with a cry of agony in our hearts, as the fragile thread of our faith is dealt with so violently. Is anyone strong enough to stay conscious through such teaching as you are receiving? Probably very few. And even they would only have a whisper of equanimity and peace amidst the screaming trumpets of their rage, grief, horror, and desolation.*
>
> ***I can't assuage your pain with any words, nor should I.*** *For your pain is Rachel's legacy to you. Not that she or I would inflict such pain by choice, but there it is. And it must burn its purifying way to completion. For something in you dies when you bear the unbearable, and it is only in that night of the soul that you are prepared to see as God sees and to love as God loves.*
>
> ***Now is the time to let your grief find expression.*** *No false strength. Now is the time to sit quietly and speak to Rachel and thank her for being with you these few years and encourage her to go on with whatever her work is, knowing that you will grow in compassion and wisdom from this experience. In my heart, I know that you and she will meet again and again and recognize the many ways in which you have known each other. And when you meet, you will know, in a flash, what now it is not given to you to know: Why this had to be the way it was."* Our rational minds can never understand what has happened. Our hearts, if we can keep them open to God, will find their intuitive

> *way. Rachel came through you to do her work on earth, which includes her manner of death. Now her soul is free, and the love that you can share with her is invulnerable to the winds of changing time and space.*
>
> *In that deep love, include me.*
> *In love,*
> *Ram Dass*

Powerful words from a great spiritual leader. Author C.S. Lewis said, ***"We read to remind us we are not alone."*** A special thanks to Dr. Wallner et al. for powerful words of inspiration, reminding us to strive to rise stronger continually.

Dr. Michael B. Grossman, DM, MSN, RN
Author, Consultant, Friend, Mentor

ACKNOWLEDGEMENT

I would first like to acknowledge and thank my spouse, children, grandson, and family for their patience and support during this book's completion. I would also like to thank my doctoral colleague, Dr. Michael Grossman, D.M, for his wise counsel about self-publishing and completing the book's foreword in record time. He is a well-respected author, practitioner, and consultant, and an invaluable mentor and friend.

By the time this book is published, it will be the second in the **Rising Stronger Series™**. The first book in the series: *Rising Stronger: Living, Loving, and Leading from a Seat of Gratitude* is my memoir (February 2019). Ever since, and because of the overwhelming response to my first attempt at self-publishing, I have had a *strong* desire to create a series to help different population segments develop their blueprint for Rising Stronger™.

The second book in the **Rising Stronger Series™** is possible through contributors, writers, and editors' collaborative efforts. This book's stories, told by amazing women I have known for 20-43 years, act as conscious awakenings of love and heartbreaking reminders of life's tragedies. These women will forever connect by invisible badges of bravery, resilience, and tenacity. They live by unquestionable energy and passion for keeping the faces of their children alive. In doing so, they share how they have been managing their lives after enormous losses.

Let me take time to pay homage to the women who agreed to share their stories of Rising Stronger™ after losing a precious child. I thank them for their courage and willingness to help others to heal after losing a loved one. It is not for fame or fortune that these women have agreed to share their stories. It is because they have a strong desire to help others struggling with similar situations. The courage demonstrated by the contributors in allowing readers into their lives indicates their desire to live beyond the heartbreaking experience of losing a loved one. Recognizing that there is nothing they could have done to prevent the events is a way of acknowledging a desire to heal. By writing their stories, they express their willingness to keep *Rising Stronger™*.

I am in no way a grief expert. However, like our contributors and you, the reader, my knowledge of the topic is pragmatic due to the loss of my grandparents, father, brother, best friend, and other close relatives and friends. Over the years, I faced near-death experiences with my two children. I experienced one child being read his last rights three times in one week, just after his eighteenth birthday. I am grateful that he overcame that obstacle. I held my seven-month-old child in my arms while he gasped for breath in a hospital in Kingston, Jamaica, while I wailed for help. He was immediately placed in an oxygen tent to save his life.

Additionally, if you have ever been in a situation where adult children around you are making poor, detrimental decisions, you may understand my obsession with grief. If you are a mother terrified of losing a child, perhaps this book can explain the importance of seeking help before it is too late. Do not get me wrong. People whose children have had near-death experiences or fearful of losing children due to their poor choices are unmatched to parents *who have lost a child.* Like Dr. Grossman emphasized, *"it is not a competition."*
These collective experiences help us to realize our vulnerabilities, encouraging us to approach the topic of grief delicately and cautiously. Since I started collecting and editing the stories in this book, a few more of my friends, family, and "born-country" citizens have lost their children to some of the world's deadliest epidemics: cancer, murder, suicide, and heart disease. Additional news about domestic abuses, murders, and murder-related suicides are epidemic proportions and extremely disheartening in and outside of the country. My dear sister-in-law lost her brother just days after this book was formally published, and the family is in a state of shock. These families have a difficult road ahead of them.

I sincerely hope that this book will bring parents and families experiencing such devastation some comfort.

Grief experts Elisabeth Kubler Ross & David Kessler propose *Five Stages of Grief*: (1) Denial; (2) Anger; (3) Bargaining; (4) Depression and (5) Acceptance (www.grief.com). The authors advise that this is not a linear process as grieving parents may experience the stages differently. By sharing these stories, we can put one foot before the other and take our healing one day at a time. This pathway is beneficial in explaining different emotions. Naturally, other contributing dimensions discussed in the body and summary of this book will dictate how one deals with grief.

Writing or editing these stories was extremely difficult because I know the parents and had met most of the children. The more complicated the novels became, the more determined we were to finish this collaborative effort. Our stories may not be new to our readers. Nevertheless, our viewpoints and increasingly *intermittent Rising Stronger™* moments may act as counsel to others.

CHAPTER 1: INTRODUCTION

Like the early experiences of many prominent authors, I have had a burning desire to write books. Not just to tell fictional stories, rather be a voyeur into the human condition. My strategy is not to judge. Instead, my goal is to seek deeper human understanding by exploring family, friends, colleagues, and clients' lived experiences. Such exploration's primary objective is to find lessons for others destined to walk similar or unfamiliar paths.

A second objective of sharing life stories includes presenting different angles to overcoming obstacles. It is about finding ways and means to swim to the surface, even when the world beneath your feet is imploding into a gorge. When we are tumbling into the chasms, and life seems unbearable, it is essential to find a limb. Persevering, striving, and enduring despite seasons of screaming, swirling, slushing into intolerable existence, requires determination and faith.

Life is so short and filled with regret that denying affection within families is ill-advised. We should not wait until we are in a predicament or dying before verbalizing and showing love for our family and friends. My maternal great-grandfather pledged his love for his wife while being swept away in a swift river of muddy water after a fierce storm in Jamaica. He thought he was about to die and found the courage to send a message via the villagers trying to save him: *"Tell Mehella, if we no meet yah, we will meet a yonder world oh."* This statement is an older version of the Jamaican dialect, translated to mean, *"Tell my wife not to worry. If I die now, it is not the end of our lives together. We will meet again when Jesus comes."* He lived well beyond that experience and never failed to express his love.

Unfortunately, not everyone has an opportunity to say goodbye. For some, there is time to plan for the departure. For others, the notice is short—scandalously sudden—distinctively loud. As you will learn in the stories within, a child's sudden passing leaves family members breathless—in a surreal state. Not everyone had a tangible branch to hang onto with the hope of meeting their loved ones on earth again.

No matter how much notice we receive, losing a loved one is tough. Grief often lingers menacingly. Mentally, some individuals, locked into an emotional prison of "Whys?" have difficulties healing. *As we knew it, life took a turn for the worst, and they reluctantly relive the moments* when it happened. We replay our actions during the last encounter we did not know would be final. Unfortunately, it was final, and there was little or no time to say goodbye.

As you read the stories in Chapters 2-9, you will realize grief has no specific measure; no blueprint for living one's life after a tragedy or unexpected passing. However, one person's story can change the path of another person's journey through the grieving process. Because of this sharing practice, support groups are so essential.

By listening to someone's experience, members realize they are not alone. Chapters 10-11 examine grief from cultural and gender perspectives and its toll on family units. Chapter 12 is particularly instructive to the suffering and organizational leaders dealing with grief in the workplace. Chapter 13 proposes support based on spiritual and faith-based practices.

If you live beyond twelve, you are old enough to read and understand this book's stories. As a reader, you cannot help feeling empathy for the women sharing the moments when time stood still—when they experienced dark days and sleepless nights. When they walked around with eyes wired shut and hearts open to the raw reality that yet another child—their precious child—departed this world way too soon.

We know not when a prudent decision to avoid traffic leads to the untimely death of two young men; a slight skid on a motorcycle due to its unexpected acceleration turns fatal; a hidden illness reveals itself one misty morning and cancer reared its ugly head; a sharp turn, perhaps to save an animal while driving home one night, is fatal; an eighteen-wheeler takes out one male adult and three male children of the same family; a man who served his country diligently is beaten to death by another in his homeland; or a woman is killed early one Sunday morning by someone she trusted, while her children slept quietly. Imagine one family losing two children 18 years apart.

In addition to the stories told in this book, countless families lost their loved ones under vicious, unthinkable, and avoidable settings. The media unveils grief in several reports of abject brutality and neighborhood atrocities. Heartache or sorrow no longer hides behind shrouds of darkness. Both the media and research indicate that homicides by close family members and partners are escalating, as are killings committed by strangers. Social media also unveils the cruel and pervasive patterns of behavior, leading us to believe that life, though priceless from bereaved parents' perspectives, is worth nothing to those who take life maliciously.

It would be remiss of me not to send a message of empathy, hope, and love to parents who recently lost a child. Some of these events occurred in ferocious and appalling settings. I have had conversations with a couple of parents whose grief is still too raw to discuss. In times like these, we listen more than speak—sometimes in the richness of collective silence. There is no band-aid or quick fix for grief. Meandering through the maze of despair requires healthy doses of courage, tenacity, and honest confrontation about how to pick up the pieces and go one without our loved ones. As you read these stories and recognize how fragile life is and how vulnerable we all are, do not forget to express love and support for those left behind.

> *"There is no "right way" to grieve for the passing of a loved one. Culture, values, personality, stage of life, and relationship with the deceased play significant roles in how people mourn their loss and celebrate the lives of their loved ones." Dr. Pauline E. Wallner, D.M.*

CHAPTER 2: "HE IS OUR COUSIN—HE IS OUR BROTHER"

By
Pauline E. Wallner (Nee, Nooks)
for my brother
Cleveland George Nooks (Fox)

At the age of seven, I met a small five-month-old baby boy in the tiny apartment I shared with my siblings and parents in Kingston, Jamaica. My father brought him home as evidence of his extramarital affair with the boy's mother, and purportedly, as a gift to my mother, who previously birthed six children. It was evident that the boy was special. He looked different, and he smelled like powder and coconut oil. His hair was straight at the roots, with puffy, bubblelike curls at the end. It was apparent that he had mixed racial genes. Though it was getting dark outside, we could tell by his hair texture and skin tone that we were not directly biologically connected. His skin was hairy and had a rusty hue, which earned him a well-deserved nickname, "Fox." Offered no explanations about his presence or relationship to us, we had differing opinions about his origins. As young as we were, we could not wrap our heads around infidelity, adoption, or foster parenting.

Besides, his light hue resembled our beloved uncle's son, and as such, some of my siblings thought our uncle was this boy's father.

However, the older siblings were sure he belonged to our father, which made him our brother. As we gently exchanged and tossed this beautiful child back and forth among us, we chanted, **"*Is we cousin, is we Breda*"**—translated to mean, *"He is our cousin—he is our brother."* Cousin or brother, we did not care because evidently, we claimed him as our own from day one. We could not help trying to understand why a mother would let this precious child go. He belonged to us, and he was a permanent part of the family. As a result, we spoiled him—he could do no wrong.

My mother treated him as her child, nurturing him as if she had given birth to him. When she ventured into the neighborhood with him, she held her head high against the backlash, whispers, and finger-pointing. Allegedly, she had somehow managed to give her husband a '*Jacket.*' *A Jacket is an old Jamaican jargon used to describe a child sired by one man and given to another as his child.* Since the child looked like neither parent, it was easy for the busybody neighbors to make assumptions and arrive at their conclusions. My mother never tried to correct their notions about her life. She did not think she should have to explain anything to anyone—it was none of their business. *"Let them talk,"* she would say. *"Who cares what they think?"* She would not dignify their ridiculous comments and meddling questions with a response. Walking down the street, she smiled as she hugged the baby to her bosom.

Despite the reasons Fox joined our already large family living in a tight space, he blended well into the family. He was a happy, rambunctious child who was always playing pranks on his siblings. He was usually the last sibling to hit the shower, waiting until his brothers ribbed him to do so. On the days when he took the initiative to go into the shower before his brothers, he ribbed them playfully by chanting, "Who is smelling up the place now?" When Fox was tired of playing, he retreated with a pencil and paper to draw large, looming caricatures for us to admire. He was always looking to brighten someone's day with his drawings.

He had a mechanically wired brain that fixed everything in sight, even the things that did not need fixing. He was talented and destined to become a breaker/fixer of things. As a child, he subscribed to Facebook mogul Mark Zuckerberg's philosophy, *"Move fast and break things—unless you are breaking stuff, you are not moving fast enough."* Slowly and surely, he reconstructed the items he broke—a radio—flashlight— simple toys. Forget early implementation of *Special*

Education—that did not help him either. What he could not do academically, he did kinesthetically. The stories in the murals indicated that he was an observer of life. In today's environment, it would be considered messy graffiti and its placement punishable as a crime. Back then, we called it a creative adaptation of life-art. The storyboards he created on paper and the walls in the community were reflective of our reggae culture.

I remember that even when we were older and I no longer lived at home, Fox visited the apartment I shared with my oldest sister. He grew into a thoughtful, compassionate young man who looked around to identify others' needs and used his artistic talents to bring joy and light to their lives. At the end of a visit, he would promise to get a painted canvas for us next time, and sure enough, he would bring the right blend and color scheme to match our walls. The pictures were neatly wrapped in plastic paper to prevent them from getting wet on the way to visit us. We framed them and hung them in the living room for all to see. We were so proud of him.

As Fox grew older, it was evident that academia was just not his calling. He neither had the interest nor the stamina to sit for long hours in a classroom. He became bored quickly, and while the teachers tried to get "blood out of stone," he wandered off to an imaginary place filled with cartons. He could not wait to develop and expand his craft. Any blank surface he encountered, he painted a story from his imagination. The pictures often depicted lifestyle, culture, and events of the late 80s and 90s. His talent was well beyond his years. Somehow, he could visualize and illustrate what others could not. What he lacked in academic prowess, he made up for in his artistic abilities.

Cleveland loved his brothers and spent a lot of time growing up and as a young adult. In his early twenties, he was an attractive young man who dressed well, was fun to be with, and was incredibly talented. Naturally, Fox attracted many young ladies' attention and could not seem to find the "One." As the older siblings migrated or moved into their adult lives, some marrying early and settling down, Cleveland tried to form his circle of friends. Unfortunately, he did not always make wise choices. Allegedly, he was experimenting with marijuana and perhaps other hallucinogenic drugs. When confronted with this rumor, he vehemently denied it, and, if it were true, he covered his tracks very well. His older and younger brothers, who always looked out for him, had no reason to believe that he had chosen that path. However, to be sure, several attempts were made to acquire counseling services for him about the dangers of drug use. He always believed that he did not need counseling. In his mind, since there was no problem, recovery was not a concern.

One day, I was sitting at my desk in Stamford, Connecticut, when the telephone rang. It was one of my brothers crying and mumbling something. I was not quite sure what he said though I could hear the name "Fox" and "Cleve" when his tone changed from base to soprano. I was transformed back to childhood as I wondered what the hullabaloo was all about. It was undoubtedly about Cleveland—he had died suddenly. I am not sure what I said next. I heard this annoying, gut-wrenching wailing coming from somewhere. I looked around to see if others could also hear the commotion. A colleague came over and could not get anything from me. I kept thinking, who the heck is making all that noise? "It must be bad news," my coworker said. "She is distraught." It was only when another colleague said, "I don't know why these people can't deliver bad news outside of work hours" that I realized the wailing was coming from deep inside of my stomach. Realizing it was not fair to my colleagues to be that upset at work, I quickly left the office and drove home in despair. I needed space to process the news I had just heard. Figuratively, my *cousin, who was also my brother*, passed away only a few minutes ago. He had a "flu-like" cold and did not think anything of it. I do not suppose smoking marijuana and other poisonous substance helped either. I know that he had agreed to accept counseling his brothers arranged after much pleading. He was drug-free for about a year before imprisoning himself into old habits. Supposedly, and because others had died after ingesting poisonous drugs, a rumor suggested Fox might have been a victim of a similar experience. If that were the case, his immune system could not fight the cold or sore throat that led to meningitis—his formal cause of death.

As I wrote in my previous book, "That ("sh...t.") comes with many broken promises and lethal outcomes." (Wallner, 2019). I have not tried any addictive practices that imprison the soul. However, I have seen others who suffered through that experience—a sad epidemic with severe outcomes. Cleve was told on several occasions to go to the doctor, and he lingered. Like many young people today, he was not thinking of the consequences of taking the flu lightly. His illness was worse than he thought, and what could have been treated by simple antibiotics was left to decay in his throat, leading to meningitis and death.

A thousand "what ifs" came into my mind during the next few hours. If I had stayed in Jamaica, would he still be alive? Would he have listened to me if I told him to see a doctor? He was an adult and made his own choices. I kept thinking, "He would have listened to me....." No, he would not. Smiling from the corner of his mouth, he would make promises to go and would not go. This behavior is typical of many people in the neighborhood back then. They believed in homeopathic treatments, and no number of warnings swayed them from that mindset.

The second phase of the mourning was anger with Fox for allowing this to happen. My siblings and parents were inconsolable as this should not have happened. By then, we were nine strong, and we looked out for each other. My parents were divorced, and thank God, and there was no more bitterness in their relationship. There were multiple conspiracy theories about his passing. Urban truths welded with lies did not help how we felt as we planned the funeral for Fox's untimely death. Those of us who were outside the country at the time traveled home to join our parents and siblings who were home.

The funeral service, held in the church our father attended, had standing room only. Busloads of people left the village to pay their last respects. On the way to the church in August Town, Jamaica, the buses passed the many walls with Cleve's artistic aptitude. The walls shined brighter as if saluting the boy's memory. He grew to be 26 years old. He had no children on record, yet his nieces and nephews never get tired of hearing stories about him. The village paid tribute to "Fox" in multiple ways. He was larger than life and always extremely positive. Even if he disagreed with you, he found ways to put a positive spin on every conversation. He had a unique style of laughing, talking, and teasing at the same time.

Accompanied by my siblings, I read the Eulogy. I could not help seeing his siblings from his biological mother in the left pews, the siblings from our mom and dad in the right pews. However, there was no doubt whose child he was. It was the woman who hugged him in the middle of the night when our father placed him into her arms at five months old. It was the woman who begged no thanks because her love for him and his siblings never failed. We miss him and still include him in our ancestry. We are grateful for his presence in our lives, regardless of the circumstances. God makes no mistakes—he was where he needed to be. We still laugh about the pranks he played on us and the fables that confirmed his name: "Fox."

Cleveland would have been 52 years old this year. Although the pain gets duller each year, moments when we reflect on his journey—like writing this chapter—cause our eyes to well up and our hearts to break. The pain does not go away. We just find ways to cope. Through faith and the promises of a loving God, we hope to see Cleveland and our loved ones when Jesus comes. Keep Rising Stronger™.

> *"Trust in the Lord with all your heart, and do not lean on your own understanding. In all your ways, acknowledge him, and he will make your paths straight."*
> *[(Proverbs 3:5-6 NIV)]*

CHAPTER 3: SURVIVING GRIEF IS A CHOICE

By
Annette M. Nalty
Mother of
Corey O'Neal Nalty

May has always been a wonderful month in our home. It brings warmth to suppress the chill of winter and prepares us for the heat of summer. The trees regain their leaves, and the fresh grass springs a beautiful delicate green. May is a time to plant our vegetable garden, prune our fruit trees and insulate our flower beds beneath the annuals that yield beautiful flowers. In May, we will celebrate Mother's Day, birthdays, anniversaries, births, and, sad to say, days that will forever be painful for us.

The call came at 12.30 a.m. on a Sunday. Sundays have always been unique. It was customary for us to attend church services early to mid-morning. Afterward, we would spend time hanging out at home, separating for various events, or having family dinner. This Sunday morning, however, we were away from home. We traveled to Miami to visit family and to hang out for a couple of days. Our children were grown, and though we had two adult children living at home, we were semi-empty nesting. The phone ringing at that hour of the morning might be abnormal for some families, except our kids knew we stayed up later the nights when we visited family and friends. Besides, I spoke to my eldest only an hour before, and he must be calling me back with a question. The constant ringing of the phone sent an immediate panicky alert. We had three boys in America, and our elderly parents lived in Jamaica. When the phone rings, we answer it, regardless of the time. "Who could be calling?" I thought. "What is the matter?" I wondered.

"*Hello?*" I answered with a somewhat tentative and apprehensive voice. Jordan, my youngest, quickly responded and said, "Mom, someone wants to talk to you." The next voice, stoic, trained to deliver bad news, identified himself as Sargent 'Something or Other' and uttered the words that all parents dread: "*Your son, Corey, has been in an accident.*" It is one of those moments when the world stands still. When sounds no longer echo in the background—when the truck that thundered past a few seconds ago, with the lingering, rumbling sounds of an engine, suddenly fades into the night. The place is suddenly dry. *It* appears as if all the air retreated, and you feel an emptiness. When nothing seems normal as you wait to exhale the tightening breath deep inside your lung, and you gasp for air. A million questions flash simultaneously through my mind. The question I want to ask is the one I am most afraid of asking: "Is he alive?"

I suddenly realized that the caller was still mumbling instructions. They could not tell us anymore on the telephone—we had to come to the hospital. That was our cue that this was no minor accident. They would have told us to go and get him. I looked to my husband for answers, and he expressed what I could not: "This is serious," he said. I called the hospital—still no information. It took us five seemingly endless hours to drive home to Ocala from Miami. We picked up our son, Jordan, and went to the hospital in Gainesville, Florida. No one spoke—no one could. We were all afraid to vocalize our thoughts—that the unthinkable was possible. <u>Upon our arrival at the hospital,</u> a doctor confirmed the unimaginable. Our Corey was no longer with us. At 12:50 a.m., on Sunday, March 15, 2011, he took his last breath. It was a goodbye whispered to strangers from a heart filled with love and regret. It was a wistful peace only achieved upon exhaling one's last breath.

Departure is another moment when the world stands still—when the noisy thunder beating against the closed door of my chest begs for sweet relief. Out of the corner of my eye, my husband, our family's bedrock, was struck with grief. I saw him put his hands over his face and double over. I saw the tears bubble up into Jordan's eyes and spill over, leaving tracks on his face. I could not move due to the heaviness in my heart and legs. I said nothing. The numbness of my vocal cords and my body did not permit me to speak, and I could not respond to the news. I was too disoriented to speak—cry—or move. I did not call—I could not. All this happened in the same moment as we tried to absorb the earth-shattering news.

The doctor offered his condolences, *"Take as much time as you need,"* he said and left us to our disbelief and grief. A Social Worker came in to go over the *'what comes next'* matters. "Do you want to see him now?" she asked. "Who can we help you contact?" "Where do you want to send the body after the autopsy?" Wait one minute. What the heck is going on? Did I hear her right? "THE BODY?" Time stood still until that moment. It is only then that we landed back from our places of disbelief. As if suspended on a fishing rod, clawing for freedom to get back into the water where it was safe, we landed suddenly on the floor, flat on our feet. Before the message, we were hopeful. Before we had confirmation, we prayed for grace. Mentally dragging ourselves back into that room, the reality of our immense loss was unbearable. She talked— we stared—not offering much in terms of responses to her queries. We each were conscious only of being in our place of increasingly overwhelming numbness. We did not have a name for it yet. We were still processing the events of that morning—still processing the news that our Corey was gone from this life.

Corey had been our 'better to ask for forgiveness than permission' child. He had a very expansive personality—he never met a stranger. He was always bringing strangers home with some story that they needed a place to stay or needed bus fare to somewhere. That inclusive personality came in handy to a United States Air Force brat who relocated every few years. He was a natural athlete with a big heart and a generous spirit. As a child, he was not particularly good at competitive sports because he was always concerned about losing the game. He was a gifted writer with a *great* laugh and an irreverent sense of humor. He loved video games, computers, and music. It was fascinating to observe his excitement during and after he developed various soundtracks on the computer. Some of my friends professed that his music was extraordinarily aerobic and fun.

Rarely was he seen without a set of drumsticks in his hands as a teenager. They were all over the house, seemingly multiplying daily. He was great with kids. There was a ten-year difference between him and his youngest brother, Jordan. However, when Jordan was in elementary school, his friends loved to visit the house as Corey had them running around and laughing with an odd, rambunctious game. Corey helped Jordan's friends with homework, and his patience was admirable. Corey's compassionate demeanor said a lot about who he was as a child and as a man. He had an autistic cousin (Brian), and they had the most fantastic relationship. When Brian refused to get dressed or do some other task, a call from Corey to his "Bri-Guy" would accomplish wonders.

Corey served in the US Navy. A few years earlier, he met a young lady who could not hear and relied on sign language to communicate. He took sign language so that he could share it with her. Sadly, she too was lost in a traffic accident. He had been devastated. Corey had been diagnosed with Bipolar Disorder.

> *According to the National Institute of Health, Bipolar Disorder is a "chronic or episodic (which means occasionally occurring and at irregular intervals) mental disorder" (www.nih.gov).*

He had a few years when life was a real struggle for him. He worked hard with his counselors and doctors to find the medication and treatment program that worked for him. With their help and sheer determination, he had his disease under control. He went back to college—had a job—and had just met another young lady. He and his brothers were planning a bike trip around Europe. Then came May 15, 2011.

As a teenager, he told us that he had a dream where he saw his headstone with two dates. He could read the birthdate but not the other date. However, he realized that the different date meant that he was not yet thirty years. I am not sure if he dwelt on that dream or if it was just a forgotten event. He lived with gusto, embracing life in every which way—touching others' lives in remarkable ways. He packed a lot of living in his twenty-nine years, four months, and eleven days. We are eternally grateful for his time with us.

As I reflect on the subsequent days, nothing was clear during the few weeks or even months after that May morning. Life back then involved a flurry of activities—notifications, funeral/memorial preparations, and legal stuff. All that sticks out from that time is the unbelievable *VOID*. How could he be gone forever? I spoke to him a couple of hours before the phone rang. How is it that I will never hear that voice again or see that fantastic smile? The air around me was like thick soup, and it took supreme effort to move my limbs or even lift my head. I went back to work, smiled, and said the right things. But each morning when I awoke, I felt an all-consuming sense of dread enveloping me, unwelcome as a woolen blanket on a hot summer day.

I found it difficult to pray. I was mad at God. How could he take him now that he was getting his life together and reaping the benefits of all his earlier struggles? My conversations with God, or dare I say my raging, during that time, went something like this, "You lost your son too, so you should understand—why my son—why now?" He was getting ready to live an extraordinary life. Grief does strange things to people, and each reacts differently. I could not use the word "*DEAD*" when speaking of Corey. I learned all the euphemisms—passed away—did not survive—departed, etc. It has been eight years and eight months, and I still cannot use that word. To me, it is so final—harsh and unforgiving. I know he is gone, yet speaking it out loud makes it too much of a reality.

It was also interesting to see how people reacted to someone who is grieving. Some would hug me and say, "He is in a better place," or "God needed another angel." In my mind, I was thinking, "I don't care. I need him here." Others avoided me altogether because they did not know what to say. I understood that people just wanted to offer comfort and did not know what to say. Still, others just acted as if nothing happened. Those people irritated me the most as it seemed they were discounting the precious life of my child. But again, I realize that it is difficult to know how to console someone on such a significant loss. Having walked the plank, I now have a better understanding that, in general, people mean well. There are no words sufficient to console a grieving parent. However, merely acknowledging the loss with "I am sorry" goes a long way.

Someone from my church suggested a support group called *Compassionate Friends*. The first visit was difficult, and I left before the end of the meeting. Maybe it was too early—six weeks after. There were people there who were still struggling two and three years after losing their loved one. I panicked as I realized that I could not continue feeling the way I was for another two years. One thing stuck with me with little uncertainty—two more years of this numb existence was too long. One of the ladies sharing at the meeting said that ***surviving grief is a choice***. I do not know if I decided that very same night. I knew, however, I had no choice but to *Keep Rising Stronger*. He had a conquering, compassionate spirit and would want us to thrive beyond our grief. Corey embraced life through its ebbs and flows, and there have been many. He would console us and encourage us to keep rising stronger. Corey was an overcomer and a beautiful soul. He would want us not to give up or give in—to place one foot before the other and walk by faith.

Handling grief is a personal journey. In the early days, I wanted to know everything about the accident. "Was he conscious?" "Did he suffer?" I requested a copy of his autopsy report, hoping to get some glimmer of understanding. I read that report so much I almost had it memorized. Corey's formal cause of death was: ***Atlanto-occipital Dislocation (AOD).*** Those words became flashing neon lights in my mind—a heavy metallic mantle on my head. I read the police report. I conducted several types of research to get familiar with all the medical terms listed in the autopsy. I visited the location of the traffic accident.

> *I got permission from the city to install a road marker in Corey's memory—a place to stop for a visit on my way home and a place to be reminded of the boy that went home too soon.*

I would fall asleep on Saturday nights just to wake up at about 12:00 a.m. and watch the clock until 12:50 a.m.—the time he was officially pronounced lifeless. In the end, however, none of this eased the enduring sense of loss.

It was not easy—this "surviving grief" thing. Grief came in waves. One day I think I am doing OK, all things considering, then the next, I am all crumbles. With the best of intentions, sometimes the waves were too much to handle. Small things would trigger these moods like the crashing, sucking, dragging sound of an unforgiving tsunami—ready to drag us all into its swelling, tasteless drama. The smell of his favorite fragrance or seeing a car like the one he drove were some of the simple triggers that caught me off guard. I went to pieces one day after passing a Verizon store, the last place we visited together.

The things we took for granted before Corey's passing became monumental *track*-stoppers for the next couple of months.

The challenge was not to stay in that space, figuring out how to claw back from that dark place. For me, it was to remember the happy times. The times when his mouth opened into a wide grin and his eyes curled into pockets that printed dimples into his strong, handsome ebony face. Corey was a serious music lover. That boy loved music. He had an eclectic taste in music and a particular love of Queen and 80's music.

> *"I played and sang to the masterful arrangement of Queen's "We Are The Champions." That became an uplifting activity for me on days when darkness engulfed me like an endless storm; grief tempted blindness to any sign of joy."*

Queen would cringe at my screeching version as I butchered their masterpiece at the top of my lungs, sometimes while the tears were still coursing down my face.

I think the true catalyst to my way back from the darkness of consuming grief was a dream I had. I say a dream because I have no other word for it as it was so real to me. I was lying in bed early one Saturday, about five months after that fateful May morning. In the dream, Corey walked into the bedroom and came to sit on the bed. He looked wonderful with just a little scratch under his right eye. I told him that I had three questions: (1) What happened with the accident? (2) Were you afraid? (3) Are you OK? I do not remember the answer to the first two questions. What was profound for me was his answer to the third question. *"Of course, I am alright; lots of people seem to have lots of questions for me."* We chatted companionably for a while, as was our custom. He laughed that happy, inimitable laugh and said it was time to leave. I said to him, "Last time you left without saying goodbye, and I was crushed." However, this time, he left with a gesture that was so Corey—a gesture I had seen so many times before. He half-turned and looked over his shoulder so that I could see that famous smile, nodded, and waved as he walked out of the bedroom. When I got up that Saturday morning, it seemed that I had a new lease on life. It seemed that the unwanted emotional blanket dissipated. I gave my house a good cleaning—something I had not done in months—and I went for a long walk. I have no idea what the significance of the dream was. I know that it made my spirits soar that morning—something that I did not think was ever possible again. Now I am by no means saying that after that day, it was all happiness and joy. But I am saying that I could see myself starting to make progress after that day—to start living again.

While walking through grief is a personal journey, it also helped me not to isolate myself. We had a wonderful group of friends who circled the wagons around us. For the first few weeks, we found it challenging to be in the house. Our friends arranged barbeques and rotated, sending us invitations for dinners or just evenings out at their homes. Their understanding was like a welcome rain on a parched day. My good friend Carmen would get me each morning before work and on weekends, and we would walk. The long quiet walks were good for the body and quieted my soul.

I eventually went back for a few visits to *Compassionate Friends*. Eight years later, I still attend the group's Candle Lighting Memorial Service each December and Butterfly release each May. Through the group, I met a wonderful couple who had also lost a son and founded a memorial park to help families deal with a child's loss. My involvement with this fantastic group of people was a real gift. We understood each other's collective yet uniquely individual journeys. We talked about our children without judgment—sometimes other people were uncomfortable with the subject. We shared our struggles, our triumphs—laughed, cried together, and of course, broke bread together.

> *"Also, my involvement with the Memorial Park gives me a sense of purpose and a tangible way to honor Corey, ensuring that he is not forgotten."*

That year of "firsts" was tough. The first birthday, Thanksgiving, Christmas, and New Year after his passing were not easy. Our family surrounded us again, and we had lots of company for Thanksgiving, Christmas, and into the new year. I survived Thanksgiving and Christmas, but when that clock turned over to 12:01 a.m. on Jan 1, 2012, I lost it. I did not see it coming until I heard a wailing, a gut-wrenching wailing—a few moments before I realized that the sound bubbled up and spilled from deep within me. The realization hit me. This year and subsequent ones would be without our Corey. May 2012 was also a challenge. Once the calendar page turned to May 1, that familiar feeling of dread came creeping back again. I started my countdown—fourteen days to live—thirteen days. My amazing, lifelong friend altered her travel plans to ensure that she would be with us to help us navigate what she knew would be our most challenging "first." But even her loving presence did not deter that feeling of dread from growing more profound and spreading like a dark stain over my psyche. I felt like I was suffocating, and I could not do anything to stop that day from arriving. Then the day dawned—

unchallenged—untamed—interrupted only by the anxiety developing deep inside my spirit.

I kept breathing though—in—out—in—out—putting one foot before the other until it was May 16. Each May since I have carried out this unconscious countdown. However, that foreboding that had accompanied the initial years has lessened as the years passed. I also run a 5K each year on Mother's Day in Corey's memory. I would like to think that he runs beside me cheering me on during moments when I feel tempted to quit. I imagine that, like so many other occasions when he accompanied me to the various fund-raising events, he was there applauding my resolve to keep rising stronger.

Grief is an unforgiving, inconsiderate companion. No one willingly vies for its presence. However, having been forced to walk with that unwelcome partner, I learned a few things. I realized that I could survive anything. My unimaginable, worst fear came to pass, and I am still here. Albeit even a work in progress but I am surviving. I am learning to be courageous—not to shy away from this gripping, challenging, and exciting world because of my grief. I embrace opportunities to do/learn different things, especially as they relate to my husband, sons, family, and friends. The moments I spend with my loved ones are immeasurably treasured. "Don't sweat the small stuff" is a famous adage. And I am learning to notice and celebrate the small things.

> *I frequently hear about "living your best life," and I am trying to do just that, realizing that my idea of my best life may be different, and that is okay.*

Our mental precursor has two time-capsule dualities, "*Before Corey and After Corey.*" He is still an integral part of our lives. Each year on his birthday, we release twenty-nine white balloons to celebrate each year of his life. We do not avoid his name in conversations. You see, Corey had no children. It is up to us to keep his memory alive while we are still here. He will always be with me—that his departure from this life cannot break the bond. We still have intimate conversations on various issues and decisions. Of course, it is a matter of "What would Corey do or say about this situation." Someone once pointed out that there is a word for people who lose their parents—an orphan. There is a word for a person who has lost a spouse—a widow or widower. There is no definitive word for a person who has lost a child. I expect that this is not the natural order of things—it is an unnatural state for a parent to lose a child. However bizarre this state, it is a reality for so many of us. Recognizing that fact, I have to learn to survive and thrive as I honor the memory of our beloved Corey.

Reflection Exercise

Corey Nalty's Story

After reading Annette Nalty's experience in this chapter, please reflect and respond to the following questions:

Question/Statement	Reader's Response
1. How can you help yourself deal with the emotional strains that grief brings?	
2. How can you help others deal with the emotional strains that grief brings?	
3. List and describe the physical activities you can start or continue doing to gain physical, emotional, and spiritual strength.	
4. Make a list of similar support groups in your area that you can attend.	
5. As you review your child's **teenage/adult** experience, is there a grassroots volunteer organization, community advocacy, high school, or college *you believe can benefit from a scholarship in your child's name?*	

CHAPTER 4: THE HEART OF A MOTHER

**By
Valdete A. Paiva-Cargill, Chef
Mother of
Melanie K Cargill-Barbour**

Ever since I was a little girl, I dreamt of being a mother. In my estimation, it was an achievable goal—a simple and unpretentious little girl's dream. By the time I was twenty-five, I was still single. My hope started shrinking. But as usual, God has a way of setting things straight. Out of the blue, one spring day in 1968, I met prince charming at my doorsteps. At the time, I lived in Allston, Massachusetts, now recognized as an official neighborhood of Boston and an adjacent city to Brighton.

In those days, we did not have formal matchmakers that I knew of, and for those who can recall, we were a long way from the Internet phenomenon and online dating. It was unusual for someone to meet a life partner at home, and we connected right away. I was ecstatic—now my dreams had possibilities, and the main ingredient—a real-life prospect was standing in front of me. My head was spinning, and my heart raced in anticipation of getting to know him. We arranged a series of meetings filled with interesting chit-chat, heightening my tension of realizing a childhood dream.

At the age of twenty-nine, I received the gift of a very handsome baby boy. To me, he was flawless—the ultimate consummation between two people who met not too long ago on a doorstep. Two people were merging their dreams into one. Their aspirations for their future life were comparable to none. I was thrilled and almost unrecognizable with joy. Although we all know what newborns look like, no one could sway my confidence about the future of my firstborn. He had red blotches, a wrinkled face, a bald head, and bubbling sounds that indeed announced his arrival. Happiness and joy filled our lives, and we fondly nicknamed him "Turkey Baby" because he was born five days before the thanksgiving celebration that year. A wonderful gift from God.

Six years went by, and I got baby fever again. By then, I was thirty-five years old. In my mind, my biological clock was ticking, and naturally, I felt this was my last chance. To my surprise, it was a girl—a companion to my son who was now six years old and a happy balance in our home. Yes, she too had wrinkles, red spots, a bald head, and a diva personality. Unlike her brother, this child was vastly different. She announced her presence every chance she got as if she was in a hurry to experience life beyond the safety of the womb. She was very demanding, curious, and very vocal. She was well-prepared to face the world. On the other hand, I was less prepared for her sauciness, which she delivered with a perky defiant look.

My daughter was about three years old, and her brother was ten when fate disrupted our lives. The man I met on my doorstep so long ago consented to the calls for freedom and stepped through the door for the last time. Divorce knocked at my door, and reluctantly I had to open it. Divorce is harsh, disruptive, and sad. As a single parent of two young children—the breadwinner—caregiver, I had no time to grieve. My babies depended on me. I could not let them down. I could feel the weight on my shoulders. Emotionally, we were a hot mess. I had to shrug feelings of hopelessness and fight like a big girl. I am smiling about that experience now. However, undergoing that challenge in the '70s was no mean feat.

We finally settled into our new routine. I put my trust in God and prayed a lot. I knew I would rise again—how and when I did not know. As my dream girl, Melanie seemed to be happy and content. Her brother, who by now was twelve years old, finally started to thrive academically and in sports. As for me, all I did was work, striving to keep up an amount of normalcy in our lives.

I have always had a passion for books, and I wanted to pass them on to my children. By age five, Melanie was reading small books by herself. In kindergarten, leadership was natural. She was never a follower—she was a leader in the making who learned quickly. In 1985, I thought it would be good to go back to Boston, where I had extended family. I decided to sell my home in Westbrook, Maine, and return to Boston. All welcomed a new beginning. So many things had happened, and we moved on without stopping to honor our emotions. Right about that time, I realized that we needed counseling. We needed an outside, objective counselor to help us through the rough patches. We had not gotten over the divorce, so we went for family therapy.

I could see the difference, especially with my son, Lance. He became more open about his feelings and making friends became simpler for him. As for Melanie, she seemed happy and made friends quickly. We also had my brother's girls, who were older than my children. It was a blessing to have them around. Melanie was five years younger than her cousin Soraia. They became close, living like sisters.

Knowing that Lance was college-bound in August 1990, the family returned to Maine in July 1990. I believed the move would provide more stability for Melanie and privacy for me. So, with Melanie's welfare in mind, I decided to return to Maine. With much prayer and evaluation, it was easy for me to choose a private Christian school with smaller classes. They promised more structure, discipline, and talent exploration for students. Pinetree Academy was an excellent choice for Melanie. As usual, she made friends quickly, and she even joined the choir. She had a beautiful voice, a gift she inherited from her father. She played soccer and participated in every activity in school. During the summer months, they enjoyed many recreational activities at the Seventh Day Adventist church camp—*Camp Lawroweld.*

I felt blessed and proud of my children. I saw how happy we became again. However, Melanie could never accept "no" for an answer. Every request or deal included a tribunal. Eventually, I learned to say "maybe" as a compromise—to alleviate various hearings—and that strategy worked. I miss those days of agreeing to disagree or going head-to-head with my daughter.

In December of 1994, during Melanie's senior year, the children's father suddenly passed away. It was a huge blow. Lance, a senior in college, came home to bury his father and spend his last Christmas at home. After graduating from Pinetree Academy, Melanie decided to attend Southwest Adventist University in Texas. Somehow, I knew she was not ready to be away from home. It was too soon after losing her father, and the suddenness of his passing left her grief-stricken. When she returned for Christmas break, she was noticeably angry about her father's death. We talked about it, but nothing got resolved. When she returned to school, she realized that she was not ready to be away from mom. She dropped out of college, found a job, and was doing well.

In the summer of 1996, she asked me if I would consider moving to Texas. I agreed, and we rented an apartment together in Fort Worth. I got a job as a nanny, and we lived together for about a year. She got a job that included traveling, and she welcomed the opportunities to do so. Eventually, she moved to Miami to be closer to her cousin Soraia and her husband. The sisters were back together again, and Melanie was thrilled. It was very encouraging to see how happy she was—life was going well.

In September of 1999, I had another strong desire to return to Maine. There is an old saying that once you live in Maine, no matter where you live after that, there is a haunting desire to return. As you recall, I left Maine on several occasions, and when I became restless, I returned to quench my wandering spirit. By now, Lance was living in North Carolina, where he went to college. He was married and had a beautiful daughter. In the summer of 2000, Melanie left Florida to come home. I was not the only one who loved Maine. Maine offered an elegant yet quiet breather—an air of tranquility designed to mend broken hearts and fences. The children and I found solace there when my marriage ended. We found comfort there when the children lost their father. I returned to Maine when I felt restless and needed to hear the quiet voices from the voluminous trees, and even more so among the bright blaze of Autumn glory. When I needed stimulant from the wispy breeze that came much too soon before the ending of one season and indeed too early before the beginning of the other, Maine embraced me with open arms. Now, it was Melanie's turn. She was heartbroken, and it was immediately evident that she was holding her little fractured heart on her sleeves. A Cuban fellow broke her heart in small pieces. Having experienced the echoing tremor of a broken heart, I understood the intensity of temporary doom.

In the fall of 2000, Melanie wanted to enroll at the University of Maine in Augusta. However, she was reluctant to commit to the long days of classroom activity and organized attempts to complete assignments. After much contemplation *and soul searching about the pleasure that freedom and a flexible schedule would bring, Melanie changed her mind.* In the summer of the following year, Melanie decided to make Bar Harbor, Maine, a seasonal workplace destination. She was an excellent bartender and had no trouble finding a job. There, amid the boisterous environment created by temporary workers, visitors, and residents, she met a young man. I thought he was somewhat pleasant, and they dated for a few years. She could see the relationship was not going anywhere as she was continually guarding her heart against yet another heartbreak.

Something must have troubled her about the relationship. It was evident that she was agitated and perhaps consoled herself on several occasions as to why she should stay in the relationship. Her increasingly restless spirit confirmed it was time to leave, and she decided to move to Boston. One Tuesday, before she moved to Boston, she went up to have lunch with her boyfriend. They met at one of the most expensive places in Bar Harbor. He was trying to win her back, and I suppose she was having none of it. She ordered the most expensive dish on the menu and later excused herself to go to the bathroom. Instead of returning to complete the succulent meal she had ordered, she took a detour and went out through the restaurant's back door. He was furiously inconsolable. When Melanie got home that evening, the only thing she told me was that he needed a lesson and "I gave it to him!" She never told me why, and I did not press her about the reason. Whatever occurred between them to bring it to this end must have been unbearable for her. She, however, felt vindicated by her actions.

In 2006, I surprised her with a mother/daughter trip to Europe. It was an opportunity to breathe, exhale, replenish our lagging spirits, and reform our bond. It was a spiritual journey of hope and love—and it was more than we expected. It was a voyage of a lifetime, and we were both over the moon before, during, and after the excursions. Some remarkable events pushed our envelopes beyond *"bucket list"* imagination. I did not know then that we were making irrevocably happy memories. Nothing could change that experience—nothing.

Paris was never the same after Melanie, and I laid claims to a surreal adventure of a lifetime. We spilled laughter in the streets of Paris, painted it with happiness, joy, and pain while retrieving an everlasting emotion of love. My love for culinary arts and gardening could not prepare me for the food and scenery we experienced. We claimed streetlamps, Eiffel Tower, trollies, and buses as our own, dashing from one scene to another, hugging each other as two children would. We removed all subtle barriers that burned deep below, and our hearts beamed while our eyes glazed over with much love and understanding. Melanie visited Pere Lachaise Cemetery in Paris, France, to pay homage to the memory of beloved American rocker and The Doors' vocalist Jim Morrison (aliases, The Lizard King, and Mr. Mojo Risin). He died, reportedly, due to congestive heart failure in Paris, France, at age 27.

How many people can claim to have personally met and taken pictures with Bono of U2 in Dublin, Ireland? We met him at the Guinness Beer Tower. He was witnessing to young children and counseling them about the dangers of drinking. Both Melanie and I had conversations with Bono, and I was happy to take pictures with him. We were ecstatic and giddy with pride about this encounter. If you have any doubts about this interchange, my Facebook page shows proof. Although Melanie did not want to take pictures with Bono, she did not object to being *photographer extraordinaire.* I think she got a kick out of the fact that I rose to the occasion and had fun with this celebrity. I also enjoyed watching her create memories. Pictures are like paintings—only they are easier to move around. One teary-eyed gaze at them can soothe old wounds, turning sadness into fond memories.

Before our European tour, Melanie was dating a young man from Northern Ireland she met in Boston. In planning for our 2006 Thanksgiving celebrations, she asked me if she could bring him home to meet me. I agreed enthusiastically, as I wanted to meet the young man who captured my daughter's heart. My sister Sophia and her husband John joined us for Thanksgiving dinner. Dinner was more significant than I first thought, as they expressed a desire to get married during dinner. I gave them my blessing while my sister proposed a short engagement. And, no, she was not pregnant! My sister suggested having the wedding at her home in Belmont, Massachusetts, and they gladly accepted.

Wanting to keep the expenses down, we invited only our closest friends—about 20 people. On December 6, 2006, Melanie tied the knot with Hugo. I knew we were in for a challenge because of a tight budget. We had only $1000 for the entire cost of the wedding. The expenditure included bridal and attendants' dresses, flowers, cake, and *everything* else needed to have a lovely, intimate wedding. My friend Joyce and I made all the bride and bridesmaids' bouquets and the groomsmen and groom's boutonnières with flowers from Sam's club. The wedding was *supposed* to be around 2 pm. Melanie showed up at 3:30 p.m. Perhaps it was her last defiant and lingering protest about giving up her freedom. She also had persistent doubts about the union.

I wish I told her to call off the wedding because I knew she was having second thoughts. In retrospect, I wanted her to adhere to her runaway girlfriend/bride instinct of the past. It is a guilt that I carry to this day. After the small, intimate ceremony, we went to a pub in Waltham, Massachusetts, for the reception. The groom invited his mother to attend the wedding, so it was good to know his family. It was around 10:00 p.m. when the couple cut the cake. After that, most of us from Maine returned home. Melanie and her husband went away for a short honeymoon.

By February of 2007, the couple moved to Maine. The timing marked the beginning of what would turn out to be a modern-day recession in America. People were quietly whispering and commiserating about tales of financial hardships. They were feeling uneasy about financial stability. Although it was not evident then, many people later got displaced from their homes due to foreclosure. America would experience one of the largest housing scandals in its history. Therefore, it was prudent for those who discerned imminent financial upheaval to merge our housing costs to save money. As such, we sensibly shared the costs of a house we rented in Freeport, Maine.

My instinct was unusually uneasy. There was trouble brewing in paradise. I started suspecting that the fairy tale was over—happily-ever-after was doubtful. His flamboyant, suave personality was fading, and he had begun to show his true colors. I was not about to let my daughter live alone with a man who had a nasty temper. At least in my home, and when I was present, he had to respect me. I started noticing little character flaws, and not wanting to upset my daughter, I kept my thoughts to myself.

Melanie's husband got a job painting houses while worked for Bank of America's Call Center. It was great that she was making good money and had a short commute between home and work. Hugo, her husband, needed to purchase a truck for work. At the request of my daughter, and in good faith, I co-signed a loan for him to finance a vehicle. This agreement proved to be a huge financial blunder. As Melanie's mother, I was an optimist who hoped for the best. However, more and more, I could see a *jealous*, irrational streak starting to raise its ugly head in the marital bond. For readers familiar with Maine's unpredictable yet foreseeable winter weather, being stranded at work or home is not farfetched. When my daughter had to spend the night at a co-worker's house because of a severe snowstorm, and he accused her of cheating, we knew it was not right. Melanie did not want to be a failure, so she kept trying.

Another bone of contention was pressure from Hugo to file the documents to receive permanent residency in the United States. However, she wanted to make sure the marriage was stable and that despite his erratic behavior, his reason for wanting to marry her was real love and not a green card. Earlier, she had no reason to believe otherwise, but with his nagging about his residency, she had become suspicious.

On Thursday, December 19, 2007, he confessed that he did not think he loved her enough. I told him that it was between them. On December 20th, I went to work and returned earlier than usual because I forgot something. To my bewilderment, Hugo was home, and he was nervously surprised to see me. I hang out for a while because I had a hunch about why he was home unannounced in the middle of the day. Hugo said he needed to get to work. After he left, I had a forewarning that he was not telling the truth. Still puzzled, I went to work, returning later to confirm the legitimacy of my unease that day.

Much to my chagrin, I received a text from Hugo telling me that he was going back to Ireland. The truck for which I had co-signed the loan was at Shaw Supermarket's parking lot in Freeport. The keys were under the seat. I immediately called Melanie and informed her of the text message I received. When she checked her bank account, he had cleaned it out, leaving zero balance. A few days before Christmas, my daughter's husband cleaned out the bank account, stealing $7,000 of her money, leaving her penniless. She made every attempt to stop him at the airport to no avail. The plane door was closed, and he was off to Ireland. The Christmas lights went dim that year.

She was sick with anger, grief, contempt, fear, and self-pity. He had poor intentions—taken it all—made *her* a mark—cowardly actions. She was sick for over a week—it was as if she was grieving someone she did not know. She questioned whether this person was a figment of her imagination. She could not reconcile his face with his heartless actions.

By the time January came around, she was feeling good enough to return to work. It took a toll on her. We were emotionally broken. It was challenging to think about rising stronger. We felt defeated—kicked in the shins with bare feet—trampled upon by a heartless coward. How would we survive this one? What lessons can we garner from this horrible *experience?* Not only did he leave me in debt, having co-signed for his truck, but he also took my daughter's money. *Once* more, our faith in God *was more significant than our pain.* I took comfort in my faith, knowing that God never fails to come through for us. My favorite scripture states, *"Be still and know that I am God"* (Psalm 46:10). We both embarked on a prayer season, and God was gracious to us. My heart was still in pain for her. Whenever I think of what happened to her, I just want to cry.

Six months went by, and Melanie had just started to pick up the pieces, reconciling her tragedy and salving her wounds with God's grace and mercy.

On July 8, 2008, Melanie found a lump in her left breast during a shower. It was the size of a golf ball. She came into my room looking alarmed. I tried to keep calm, telling *her* that the lump might be a large fat cell. My words did not match the trepidation I felt, but I knew I had to once again be a parent by using words of comfort to override her fear. We knew it was severe in our hearts, so she called her primary care doctor the next day. He said he could not see her. She called another doctor and made an appointment for that afternoon. We were both eager to start the ball rolling by getting her breast examined by a specialist. We eagerly followed all the recommendations by the doctor. The mammogram and subsequent biopsy confirmed our harshest fears. Melanie was diagnosed with a rare type of breast cancer. It was "Stage Four Breast Cancer" with only a 20% chance of survival.

It was difficult not to focus on the 80% of people who did not make it. My optimistic personality did not kick me in the side, telling me to wake up. I felt as if my body left me standing with no place to go. We did a lot of crying together. My only daughter was now considered least likely to survive this devastating disease. She had no children. I had no grandchildren from her. Despite all the challenges she faced, her plans to live a fulfilled life splashed on the white wall of fear that enveloped our furrowed brows. My plans to retire in North Carolina soon died with the news. I had to reframe my thinking and put Melanie's survival on the table. My daughter needed me, and I was not yet ready to let her go. By now, Melanie needed to be in the twenty percent—survival—life.

She called her brother to share the devastating news. After she hung up, she told me her brother was crying so hard, and her heart broke for him. She had not seen him crying like this since they were kids. I had a client that connected us with the best oncologist at Mercy Hospital in Portland, Maine. Radiation and Chemotherapy started right away. Just as we were trying to pick up the pieces and return to a usual canvas in our lives, here we were fighting a family battle that we did not anticipate or need. The harsh reality is that we were not immune. What was someone else's tragedy is now at our doorway! The cruel truth is that cancer of any kind is real—it affects everyone. We were not only voyeurs. We were not immune. We were susceptible to this unimaginable possibility—and it was here.

The fact is that the number of people dying from cancer cases worldwide is on the rise. In 2008, cancer accounted for 7.8 million deaths worldwide, and these numbers are increasing. Lung, breast, colorectal, stomach, and liver cancers lead to most cancer deaths (www.who.int). No matter how protected we think we were, we are not immune. The monster knocking at our door was ugly, unrefined, and terrifying. This boorish intruder wanted to rob my daughter of her future and me of blissfully bouncing her children on my knees. It was about to deprive my son of his sister and his children of their Auntie. Another consecutive year without a peaceful, joyful holiday. At least last year, we had someone to blame for our pain. We knew exactly where to direct our anger. This year, tears flowed down our naked cheeks. We were vulnerable—our emotions were raw—our hearts heavy—yet we were not alone. I was screaming, but there was no sound. I was raging at an intangible brutish problem for which there was no cure. Enough with the reflections—terrible news comes in phases. We were in the disbelief phase. What exactly is the next stage?

On February 7, 2009, Melanie had a double mastectomy. Her brother Lance came home, and her dad's sister, Auntie Sharon, came up from California. I am forever indebted to my sister Sharon and my son for dropping everything to give us moral support. It was an exceedingly long battle. Once again, prayer was most important. Rising Stronger was the only way to survive, and we prayed for God's help and will. If nothing else, the women in our family are serious fighters and women of faith. God stood by us, sending all kinds of help.

On October 24, 2012, I wanted to go to Boston for the day, just to clear my thoughts and regroup. Melanie's friend Rachel came to spend the day with her. When I got to Kennebunk, I got a call from Rachel for me to return home. Melanie was having a seizure. She called an ambulance to take her to the hospital in Brunswick. I turned around and got to the hospital in about 35 minutes. I knew our days were in the countdown phase. The night before, I slept in her bed with her. She was delirious, but I had no idea how bad it was. The reality is that cancer had metastasized to her brain.

Faith, hope, and prayer were our only alternatives, and we kept squeezing our eyes shut as we petitioned God for his will. We could not lose faith because we had come too far. God delivered us through many dark places and situations. We had to keep our hope alive. One of Melanie's high school friends, Michael, returned from California. He started helping out by taking her to appointments and keeping her company. He was a real blessing, and I thank God for his kindness. On November 6, 2012, Michael took her to an appointment with a pain doctor at Mercy Hospital in Portland, Maine, where she became a patient. I was heading home from work when she called me to ask me not to go home. I headed straight to the hospital. By the time I got to the hospital, I was a hot mess. I could see the concern in her eyes, and I put on a brave front. My job was to be strong, whether I liked it or not. Thinking that the hard road ahead needed no more distractions, I stopped working the following day. I had to be with my daughter. I needed to be there to hold her hands and comfort her during this challenging, unbearable time.

When children are hurt, parents are always there to share the pain and the burden. The emotional strain when a child is ill can be so overbearing. However, if my thoughts roamed on the hardships of juggling so many responsibilities, love dragged me back to the bedside of my child. This child did not feel any pain as she stubbornly emerged into the world, eager to face life and live it to the fullest. During those times by her bedside, many things became clear to me. She was always restive and eager to explore life. Now here she was, fighting for life.

I was still optimistic and hopeful for a miracle. I visited the hospital at 7 a.m. and stayed until 11 p.m. On Thursday, I asked to speak with the oncologist, Dr. Inhorn. I had to ask him the trickiest question: *"How long does she have?"* A parent himself, he carefully prepared his response. With moist, compassionate eyes, he said, "Maximum, two weeks." My world came apart—two weeks to say goodbye to my daughter? How is that possible? A parent should not be burying a child. She was my only daughter.

I called my son with the news, asking him to come home, and he made plans to be home by Wednesday. In the meantime, I had many friends coming in and out to pray with us and give us a word of encouragement. On Friday, December 9, 2012, she told me the doctors want to keep her at the hospital for the weekend. She said, "Please take me home, mom." Saturday morning, I asked for an ambulance, and by 11 a.m., we were home. I had already arranged for hospice nurses to be there to help us out. My sister Sharon, the children's aunt (my ex-husband's sister), and her daughter Beth arrived on Monday and Lance on Wednesday. My internal support system was now in place.

On Saturday, after she settled in, I asked the nurse if she could stay a bit longer, and she agreed. I called my friend Lisa to go with me to make all the funeral arrangements. I went to the funeral place in Brunswick, and the director wanted me to turn over her life insurance to him. We left that funeral home. As a faithful believer in God's guidance, even in the middle of a storm, I was confident that God would come to the rescue. Sure enough, He came through for me one more time. On Thursday, I had to do an errand in Lewiston, Maine. On my way back, I noticed a small funeral home on Lisbon Road, Lewiston, Maine. When I got back home, I called Lisa again to see if she could meet the funeral director with Lance and me. We met with Guy Doist, owner of a simple one-room funeral home. Guy was a Christian man who was sensitive to his client's needs. After picking the casket, he gave me a total price of $4,000 for everything—compared to $8.000—$10.000 proposed by the competitor. God blessed me with good friends. That night Melanie asked her brother to sleep in her bed with her, just like when they were kids. Whenever she was afraid, he would sleep in her room. The next day he told me she slept all night.

Lance had to go back home on Sunday morning, the 11th of November. On Saturday night, we all agreed to take her to Hospice, where she would have round-the-clock care. It was tough to see my little girl leave our home for the last time. Auntie went with her. I stayed behind to take Lance to the airport at 4 a.m. As soon as I dropped him off, I headed to the Hospice House in Auburn, Maine. Lots of friends continued to come to pray and to encourage us. In preparation for my daughter's death, I had to make some painful decisions. I would go to the bank to close accounts and transfer cash from one account to another. I had to do it all before she passed. On Wednesday, I asked my friend and boss, Rachel W, to come up to Auburn, Maine, to meet with Dr. Austin, Melanie's in-house physician. Time to ask the same question again, *"How long does she have?"* The answer was, "She won't be here through the weekend." Thanks to Rachel, who helped me process the response, I was able to stand on my feet. I immediately called Lance and my niece Susie to give them the finality of the news. Thankfully, they all arrived on Friday night, November 23rd. On Friday, I had to come home to make sure the hospital bed was gone and anything else that needed to go.

On my way back to the Hospice home, I stopped at TJMAXX in Auburn to pick up her funeral dress. I chose a simple black dress and a black sweater and went back to the Hospice to sit vigil. I stayed by her side all night long. At 6:15 a.m. on Saturday, I went into the bathroom to freshen up. About 6:30 a.m., my niece Beth knocked at the door for me to come out. My baby Melanie was entering into rest as peaceful and as calm as she could be.

I assured Melanie I was there. She said a faint goodbye and closed her eyes. She had the most beautiful smile on her face. As soon as she passed, I called a few friends to come over and prepare her for burial. It was symbolic that I bathe her at the end of her life. I had given her the first bath thirty-five years ago. I prepared her for the funeral home as I called the director to come for her. I had asked him not to put her in a body bag, so he brought a beautiful handmade quilt.

A traditional Brazilian burial occurs within 24 hours of death. I had no time to process her passing as I was too busy walking her through the end of her life and making sure that she had a proper burial. She was going to be buried the very next day, Sunday at 11 a.m. Visiting hours were Saturday: 4:00 p.m. to 9 p.m. I asked friends not to buy funeral flower arrangements. Instead, I suggested Poinsettias—Melanie loved Poinsettias. I went to Home Depot to pick up large Poinsettias. The clerk asked me if I was having a Christmas party. I said, "no"—it is for my daughter's funeral. She looked at me and said they are $4 each, instead of $14. Everywhere I turned, people were helping me to rise stronger. In the middle of my grief, I made a mental note that *gratitude is a must.*

Considering that the burial notice was the day before, I was grateful for the family and friends who turned out to celebrate Melanie's life. The funeral home was so crowded, and people had to wait a bit to come in. I was grateful for the dozens of calls and cards I received during this difficult time. When families grieve for their loved ones, it is the most strenuous time of our lives. I felt I had put on my autopilot demeanor and wanted to make sure everything was in place, just as my daughter would have it had she been with us. By 9:30 p.m., we returned home from the viewing. I was exhausted physically and emotionally. I went to bed to cry until it was time to get up and get ready for burial.

We went back to take her to her last residence. She had asked to be buried by Grammy Frankie, and my sister-in-law generously donated a plot at South Freeport Cemetery. When we got back from the cemetery, my dear friend Rachel was at the house. She brought over 100 sandwiches for our guests. She had the table set up and had hot water for tea and coffee. At the cemetery, about 100 people were waiting for her. I said to my sister, "It looks like the burial of royalty." She answered me, "Of course it is. She is the daughter of the King." Her memorial service was at Brunswick Seventh Day Adventist Church on Monday, November 26, 2012, in Brunswick, Maine. I wrote her a love letter instead of a Eulogy. My sister Sophia sponsored the church reception.

The most challenging road to travel is the one I took that Monday evening. I was returning home without my daughter. By Tuesday, most of our out-of-town guests returned to their respective homes, including Lance and his family. My sister Sophia's husband John and my niece Susie left right after the service. My sister-in-law Sharon stayed with me for another week. The journey without my beautiful daughter Melanie in my physical presence has been extremely tough. Each time I hear a burst of laughter or see a beautiful smile, I stop to reflect on the short time we spent together. Many parents reading this chapter may have experienced something similar and are even struggling to rise stronger.

Prayers from my church family and friends are sustaining me. I could not let go of God again because he was answering my prayers. He knew that I would love and remember Melanie forever. God's grace prevailed. When I called the funeral home about expenses, the man laughed and said, "This has never happened before. Someone came and asked to pay for the expenses anonymously." Deep in my heart, I knew who that someone was, and I remain incredibly grateful.

As for me, I am a 78-year-old-woman who puts on my big girl demeanor to comfort those who are grieving for someone. I remember and applaud the thoughtfulness of the people who stood by me through all the ups and downs. I remember the times when I question God's motive and blame every heartbreak and negative encounter for what happened to my daughter. God has a way of keeping things simple for us. From the day we are born, we start to die. I am glad that Melanie embraced the beauty of God's holy spirit even during her darkest challenges. I am happy that what some may have perceived as restlessness was an innate drive to see more in a short time. I am delighted that we went to Europe together. I am comforted that she experienced love and heartbreak. Do I have regrets? You bet I do. However, when seasons of regret approach, I listen to a soft, encouraging whisper: "*Keep Rising Stronger.*"

It has been seven years, and I still cry. I am a true testimony that the Lord brought me through this valley of light turned to darkness—back into the light. I serve an awesome God! I am seventy-eight years old and looking forward to the return of the King. I am completing a Justice Studies degree at the University of Maine in Augusta (UMA). I would like to dedicate this story to every parent who lost a child. This non-fiction narrative was most challenging yet cleansing and liberating. By sharing Melanie's life with the world, I can focus more on how she lived and not how she died. Today I can genuinely say through God's grace, I am Rising Stronger.

> *"The Lord himself goes before you and will be with you; he will never leave you nor forsake you. Do not be afraid; do not be discouraged."*
> (Deuteronomy 31:8)

Reflection Exercise
Melanie K. Cargill-Barbour's Story

Having read Mimi Cargill's experience in this chapter:

How can you help yourself to deal with the emotional strain of grief?	How can you help others to deal with the emotional strain of grief?

Reflection Exercise
Love Letter

Mimi Cargill wrote a love letter to her daughter, which she rereads to comfort her in times of loneliness. Begin today by writing a love letter to your child. Start with a couple of paragraphs.

Each time you have an emotional low or a reason to be joyful, add to the letter. Feel free to use the blank pages provided at the end of this book or use a journal. If you are in a support group or subscribe to a self-help magazine, publish your letter so other parents can gain insights into your experience.

> *"Keep breathing through the pain. It may be a while before you can speak of or to anyone about your child. When that time comes, don't hold anything back. Speak of the good, bad, and indifferent so you can help those who still have a chance to make amends." (Dr. PAULINE E. WALLNER)*

CHAPTER 5: HUGS, TICKLES, AND KISSES FOR MOM

By
Valerie M. Shelton
Mother of
Wayne Vincent Shelton

No doubt, Richard Shelton is the love of my life. We got married on June 28, 1975. We met at a party after spending a weekend in Jamaica's infamous capital. Kingston's notoriety stemmed from many urban legends in those days. Richard is from the eastern part of the Island. Back then, the chances of a northerner and easterner meeting were more likely to happen in Kingston, one of the "touchpoints" on the island. My friend was dating my future husband's friend when I met him. About four months later, I moved to Kingston. My friend had an invitation to the movie and would not go without me as her chaperone. I decided to escort her. To my pleasant surprise, it was a double date with Richard.

We enjoyed our time together as a couple, and on January 5, 1978, our first son, Wayne, was born. He was the most beautiful baby I had ever seen. He was our baby, and we beamed with joy and happiness over his birth. Much to our surprise, he weighed ten pounds. He was colicky, and being a new mother, I kept feeding him. Since his condition worsened, I called the hospital, and they recommended Woodward's gripe water. Every evening between 6:00–10:00, we had to walk around with him until he fell asleep. After a few months, he was better and thrived significantly. He was a pleasant child and a delight. He did not walk until his first birthday—truth be told, he ran on that day, using his hands to balance him.

Wayne tried to get past our disciplinary measures even at a young age. He was always getting into things and waited for us to tell him to "stop." Two years later, his sister, Stacey, was born. He was very protective of his sister. He could not address her by her name, so he asked, "What are you doing, Mommy?" "I am going to bathe Stacey," I would reply. I turned my back for a minute and returned to see him trying to lift his sister off the bed. I said, "What are you doing, Wayne?" "I am bringing "Tacey" to you," he responded.

Our son Toby came ten years after Wayne was born. The first two children and their father named our third child. Everyone wanted to ensure they had input. Subsequently, his name became Toby Marvin Anthony Shelton. That is the essence of our family.

On April 1, 1989, my husband migrated to New York City to live with his mother. Although the entire family received their permanent residency (Green-Card) in the

United States of America, it was prudent for Richard to come first and set himself up before we arrived. I had a lucrative position at Scotia Bank, Jamaica, Limited, and, as a precaution, stayed back in Jamaica for about four years. With Richard living in the United States and the added challenge of retaining housekeepers and nannies for the children, we discussed sending the children to live with Richard and his mother in Florida. Since his mother stayed home, she could take care of the children while Richard worked.

The children migrated to live with their father and grandmother in 1990 while working at the bank in Jamaica. The separation was taxing because I missed my husband and children. Although I visited often, I needed to be there full-time to provide emotional support. When I finally gave up my job in Jamaica and arrived in Florida, I did not work for about six months. After working in entry-level positions for a while, I got a job at the housing authority and stayed there until I retired twenty-three years later.

On Sunday, February 12, 2012, my son came to my home to bring me some DVDs. These were movies he had at his house that I wanted to watch. As usual, when he came, he hugged and kissed me playfully on my neck. He knows that I am afraid of my neck because this tickles me. It was his playful gesture to remind me of the undeniable bond we shared. On this beautiful Florida day, he rode his motorcycle to visit me instead of driving his car. He bought the motorbike about four months before. As I remember that day, I feel compelled to pause and share a related event two years prior.

My husband and I have three children in the order of boy, girl, boy. Wayne, the oldest, was sharing an apartment with his sister. Wayne came to my home one evening riding a motorcycle. I asked him whose bike it was. He said he borrowed it from a friend. I told him, "You know I don't like motorcycles." He said, "I know, mom, but I just borrowed it for a ride." You see, we have friends that had terrible accidents riding motorcycles. My husband's friend lost his leg, and my youngest son's friend died riding a bike. He was only eighteen-years-old and the firstborn of his family of three children.

Over the next couple of months, Wayne rode the motorcycle to our home. I kept asking him if the bike belonged to him, and he kept denying it. I asked his sister about the motorcycle. She said:

> *"Mommy, I don't know why he keeps lying to you. I told him to tell you the truth. The motorcycle belongs to him." She told him, "Mom has a feeling that the motorcycle belongs to you. Why don't you just tell her the truth?"*

He finally came and told me the truth. The motorcycle belonged to him. I was upset with him. He said, *"Mom, the reason I did not tell you the truth was that I know how you feel about motorcycles."* He enjoyed riding and was reluctant to give it up. I said to him:

> *"You know I don't want you to be a victim of the motorcycle, having some terrible accident, or even dying."*

He said, "I know, Mom, but I will be cautious." He kept riding the motorcycle, and I kept nagging him about it until after about six months, he sold the bike.

A year after this event transpired, he bought a small apartment for himself and moved in. My son worked with a cable company, and he could not park the company vehicle where he lived. As a result, he parked it at our home in the evenings, returning to pick it up in the mornings. Wayne usually picks up the work truck at 7:30 a.m., just before I start my thirty minutes commute to work. One Monday morning, he did not come to get the truck. When I got to work, I texted him, *"Hey, no work today?"* He did not reply. I called him five minutes later and got no response, so I left a message *"Call me to let me know you are okay."* I called his sister, *"Have you spoken to your brother since yesterday?"* She said, *"No, Mom."* I told her he did not come to get his work truck that morning. I texted and called and got no response. She said she would call him and get back to me. You see, I had reasons to be concerned. I communicate with my children every day. I want to confirm they are okay.

My daughter called me back saying that she did not get him, and she thinks I should check on him at his apartment. He lived five minutes from where I worked. At this point, I was too concerned. So, I went to his apartment, rang the doorbell several times, and got no answer. I entered the apartment using the key he had entrusted to me. The place was in darkness. I started to shout his name, *"Wayne! Wayne! Wayne!"*—getting louder each time. After the fourth time, I heard a groggy voice, *"Yes, Mommy."* I was downstairs, and he was upstairs. I shouted, *"Are you okay?"* He said, *"Yes, Mommy."* Mad and relieved at the same, I slammed the front door and left. I called his sister and said, *"The darn boy was in his bed sleeping."*

Wayne called me at about noon and said, *"Mom, I woke up earlier, felt tired, and decided not to go to work."* I said to him, *"You should have called me the same time you decided not to go to work to save me the worry."* He apologized and said, *"I should have called then, but I was not thinking."* I responded:

> *"You pick up your work truck every morning when you are going to work. You didn't pick it up this morning and thought nothing of it? Don't you think I would be worried?"*

He said, *"Sorry, Mom. I am so sorry. It won't happen again."* I said, *"Betta not."* His sister also rubbed him about it.

Our family has a close relationship. We talk to each other every day. If they do not call their father, he would ask me, *"You talk to your son today?* Or ask, *"You talk to your daughter today?"* We try to eat together once every week. We celebrate birthdays with a special dinner at home or go to a restaurant. We play games together: Pokeno, Kalooki, or Pictionary. We also go to the movies together. When the youngest child gets out of hand, his older brother and sister usually speak to him, helping him get back on track. If Wayne visits our home and I am not there, he calls to find out where I am. If I am with his sister, he says to her jokingly, *"Don't you know you have to check with me before you take her out."* Once a month, the family visited Cold Stone ice cream parlor and tried different flavors. Every other Friday, my son and I saw a particular McDonalds' where we each had an ice cream cone. This particular McDonald's ice cream tasted better than the rest—and trust me, we have tried quite a few McDonalds'.

My son and I did many things together, such as buying gifts for his godson, decorating his apartment, getting gifts for friends and family, etc. Whenever he is buying things for his apartment, he would come for me to go shopping with him. When he was buying sheets for his new bed, he picked up these light blue plaid sheets. It was gorgeous. I said to him, *"Don't buy that."* He said, *"Why?"* I said:

> *"The thread count is 250, and it is going to be rough against your skin when you lie down on it. You should not buy any sheet set below 300 thread count."*

He did not buy that one. He found a light blue stripe one instead that was 450 thread count. From that day forward, whenever he goes to purchase sheets, he would call to ask me, *"What's the thread count again?"* His sister decided to give him a sheet set for his housewarming gift and asked him what color he wanted. He told her blue because it was his favorite color. He reminded her to make sure the thread count was over 300. She teased him with a gentle smile, *"A little knowledge is a dangerous thing."* We all had a good laugh about that.

My son enjoyed living in his apartment by himself. It had two bedrooms and two and a half bathrooms. One day I said to him, *"Hey, you know you can rent out the other bedroom to help pay your mortgage?"* He said, *"Nope, I want to be able to walk free in my apartment, with or without clothes."*

Wayne loved to cook, and I was his taste tester. He had Tuesdays and Thursdays off from work. He called me at work on some Tuesdays and said, *"Mom stop by on your way home. I cooked something.*" He was always trying out some new recipes. Most of the dinners he prepared tasted good. Some evenings I would hang around, and we would watch a movie. His sister, Stacey, was a bit jealous and would sometimes complain: "*You are always stopping at Wayne's apartment and not coming by mine.*" I said to her, "*You work nights and sleep during the days. I don't know when you are sleeping and can only visit you on the weekend.*" Furthermore, "*Your brother's apartment is on my way home. I have to pass by my house to come to you.*"

Stacey was planning to get married in June 2012. Together with the bridal party, we visited the bridal shop. Although Wayne was the best man, he was the only person missing from the fitting. Adding to Wayne's anxiety not showing up at the fitting, we received a call from the police when we got home that they would be visiting in an hour. Since both our children were away from home, we speculated about the events.

When the police arrived, they told us to sit down. Usually, that is not a good sign, and that request heightened our anxiety. The officer explained that Wayne had an accident exiting the turnpike in Sunrise, Florida, and had died immediately. No amount of speculation, fear, or anxiety could have prepared us for this news. Nothing could have prepared us for the finality of the information—Wayne was now deceased.

My biggest fear was now a reality. I begged and pleaded with my son about the dangers of riding a motorcycle. To say we were too devastated is, to put it mildly. In 2012, there were 4695 motorcycle fatalities, an increase of 7 percent over 2011. Our son Wayne was one of them. In that same year, ninety-three thousand people received motorcycle injuries (www.crashstats.nhtsa.dot.ga).

When the police had called to say they would be visiting in an hour, we were concerned. That same day, our youngest child, Toby, was driving from Orlando, where he spent the weekend. We were not sure what had happened or to whom. The police's visit was like dragging a safety net from beneath our feet and leaving us floating in the wind. We were beside ourselves with grief. I did not know what to do or where to turn.

Stacey called to see where Toby was and told him to come straight home. For his safety, we did not want to tell him while he was driving. Sadly, before Toby could hear the news from us, he saw the announcement on Facebook. We sure wished they had allowed us to share the information with family and close friends before broadcasting it on social media.

One minute we were planning for a joyous occasion, Stacey's wedding, and the next minute, we were faced with this tragic loss. We were engulfed with the darkness and hopelessness that such horrible news brings.

Wayne's best friend came over and took me to the place where the accident occurred. I had to see where Wayne took his last breath. I kept asking to see him, but the body did not get to the funeral home until the following Tuesday. He was an organ donor, so that may be a reason why it took so long. It is comforting to know that others may have benefited from his gifts.

Toby, his godmother, and I went to the funeral home. When we saw him, it was as if he had just had a shower and was sleeping. I think that added to my state of confusion. His godmother broke down, and his brother was crying. Since I had an out-of-body experience, I could not call. I was the one consoling them. His brother said, *"It should have been me."* *"No,"* I said, *"The Lord knows what he is doing."* Surprisingly, my faith was still intact. I remained committed to my religious beliefs.

> *"The Lord loaned him to me for 34 years. I am grateful for the time he was in my charge. Now, I am giving him back to the Lord."*

For the funeral, family and friends traveled from Jamaica, Canada, and other American states to pay their respects at the church service and burial. It was uncanny to see his cousins staying at his apartment without Wayne being there. Since his passing, I have spent countless nights in my son's apartment, reminiscing about our time together. If he were here now, I would say, *"Come give me a hug."*

Although Wayne was dating a lovely young lady when he died, I did not meet her until the funeral. Wayne took his time with this young lady because she was special. He told me that he would introduce her to me later. She attended the funeral, and sure enough, I liked her. We became fast friends. Although she moved on with her life, she still stays in touch. Without faith, this would have been a tough battle for me. I was not new to grief. Anguish and sadness called me by name in a significant way the year before. I lost my twin brother, Valentine, and mother-in-law, Myrel, on the same day—December 7, 2011.

As a Catholic, I had always heard about purgatory and cleansing. I did not believe it until Wayne passed. I had a dream about Wayne one month after he died. In the dream, a family friend and I were walking. A bus came and stopped. After the bus left, I saw Wayne sitting at the bus stop. Upon seeing him, I immediately tried crossing the street to sit with him. For some reason, I could not get to him. It was as if there was a deep abyss or a valley between us, and I could not reach him. He looked clean or purified, and there was steam coming off his body. I called, *"Hey Wayne, you know I love you, right?"* He nodded twice. Still in the dream, I turned to my walking partner and said, *"Did you see Wayne over there?"* When I looked back, he was no longer there. I awoke from my dream, feeling alone with my thoughts. Wayne appeared again when his sister's daughter, my first grandbaby, was born.

On another occasion, I dreamt I was at church. Both Wayne and I were walking through the back on our way to his house. He said to me, *"Mommy, I have to leave you now."* I said to him, *"Where are you going? I thought we were walking to your house."* He repeated:

> *"No, I have to leave you now." When I looked into the sky, I saw the light—Sacred Heart with a ring of fire around it—and a bright light shining down. He then said, "Goodbye, Mommy," as he moved towards the light.*

I woke up feeling a certain level of calmness and peace after that dream.

We knew that Wayne would not want us to postpone Stacey's wedding, so we went ahead as planned. He was always looking out for his siblings, and we knew he would like her to be happy. We did not replace his role at the wedding party. When it was time for the best man to enter the church and the reception, we announced Wayne's name and paused to recognize his spiritual presence. Although he was absent physically, every person present could imagine his infectious smile, boundaryless presence, and upbeat demeanor. I imagined my beautiful son Wayne giving me a firm hug, snuggling my neck, and kissing me on the cheeks. We allowed visualization and love to rule our decisions that day, and we celebrated Stacey's day with enthusiasm, pride, and passion.

We are comforted in knowing that we will meet again someday. Wayne's accomplishments were monumental, having lived only thirty-four years. He was independent yet systematic in his approach to life. He knew what he wanted, and he went after it. Historical events, now narrated as *"before Wayne's or after Wayne's passing,"* help us keep his memory alive. I miss the bear hugs and tickles on my neck. I am comforted in knowing that Wayne genuinely loved his family and friends. We are lucky to have had him in our lives, and I am grateful for the quality time together. Time is one of the best demonstrations of love—he loved his family abundantly.

Since Wayne's passing, I visit his resting place on the 12th of every month to sit and speak to him. On the anniversary of his death, the family visits him at the graveyard. We say a prayer and write endearing messages on balloons before releasing them into the clouds. I believe that God does not give you more than you can bear.

> *"You will never forget your loved ones. Your children will always be in your heart. You will overcome every challenge that you face, no matter how difficult."*

Have faith. Cry if you must. During times when I feel sensitive, I just cry. Embrace your faith. Live in the moment and be useful to your family and friends. Keep Rising Stronger™.

> *And teaching them to obey everything I have commanded you. And surely, I am with you always, to the very end of the age."*
> *Mathew 28:20*

Reflection Exercise

Wayne Shelton's Story

Valerie shared a remarkable story of faith. What actions have you taken to build and sustain relationships with spouse, children, siblings, or grandchildren after the significant loss of a child?

Your Spouse (if applicable):
Your Children (if applicable):
Your Siblings (if applicable):
Your Grandchildren (if applicable):

CHAPTER 6: TIME TO SAY GOODBYE: "MY REBIRTH"

By
Hyacinth Blake, RN, MSN, CCRN
Mother of
Renée Mishia-Gaye Williams

The millions of people who visit the tourist resorts in St. Ann, Jamaica, each year are not as familiar with its outskirts and mountainous curves that weave far above the ground into the sky. Back then, the winding, narrow dirt paved roads in the mountains giving way to the bushy precipice were *treacherous* to visitors. Yet, to the natives, like me, it was navigable, and *it was* home. I was born and grew up in the lush, green hills of St. Ann. In those days, people did not measure economic standards in units or dollars. And if it were so, we would be considered well below the poverty level as measured in the United States. One thing for sure, we were happy. Our parents loved us and never failed to instill a way of life and practice of unconditional love inside and outside the home. I attended high school in Brown's Town, St. Ann. Like many teenagers who grew up in the rural areas, migration to Kingston, the capital of Jamaica, had the promise of bright lights and lucrative job opportunities.

My entrance into the metropolis of Kingston was not without its trauma and drama. I was young and naïve in my outlook on life. Having lived a sheltered life in St. Ann, I was unprepared for the temptations I experienced in Kingston. I had to learn fast. There is an adage that reads, *Kingston kills some emotionally and others physically*. While I was unable to manage the former premise, I had to get my wits about me so that the latter would not be my outcome.

It was during this phase in Kingston that I met and married my first husband. It was not long before I received an unbelievably awesome gift of love. It was a package that traditionally took nine months to develop. It was a baby girl, and we named her Renée. A quick search on the Internet revealed the unconscious yet spiritual intent of our daughter's name. Renée is the French form of a Roman name, *Renatus*, translated to mean, reborn, or born again.

Renée's birth did not come without its fair share of anxiety. During a routine visit in the last few weeks of pregnancy, the doctor could not detect a heartbeat. Subsequently, I had an emergency cesarean section. Thank God we were able to save our baby's life. After the surgery, I did not see Renée for two days. I had to rely on her father, family, and friends to describe Renée's appearance, hue, smile, and mannerisms. The usual fears and anxiety coursed through my brain. Was she normal? Did she have the correct number of fingers and toes? How did she look? When I finally had my first glimpse of Renée, I was relieved and happy.

> *She was the most beautiful baby that I had ever seen. Later I was discharged from the hospital, and we took baby Renée home.*

I was young, inexperienced, scared, and skeptical about how I would care and provide for this baby. Renée, in her first year of life, did not sleep during the night. I remember sitting up with her in my arms, tired and nodding off, while she just laid there looking up at me. I got through the first year, then the second, and the third year. By now, the breakdown in the marriage was apparent. Friends and family members tried their best to be supportive.

On the other hand, I saw the breakdown as a personal failure. I kept most of what was happening in my life to myself. I remember writing in Renée's first photo album: "You light up my life."

> *Looking back, this child was my beacon of hope, a reason for living, and an opportunity for rebirth.*

Unfortunately, two things occurred shortly after Renée's birth. The marriage fizzled, and what looked like a simple health condition mushroomed into a severe medical condition that needed advanced treatment. Renée and I migrated to Florida in 1983, and there is no easy way to say this—life was increasingly hard in the United States, and more specifically, Florida. I thank God every day for my sister Florence who helped me in every way she could.

Renée started school in Florida and went through the school system from Kindergarten to university. She attended the University of Southwest Florida in Tampa. She later returned home and completed the Registered Nursing (RN) program at Edison College in 2011. She was on the night shift at the hospital where I worked. She was a compassionate and considerate nurse who cared for her patients and peers.

> *Renée was young, intelligent, and beautiful. She was introverted at times and outgoing other times. With a charming smile that lit the room from a far-off, she lived life on her terms.*

I would be lying if I painted my daughter as a saint. Although she did not crave the limelight, she had a selective group of friends, and she loved to socialize. Though somewhat reserved, she was a spontaneous and unique individual who enjoyed Karaoke with friends. In her younger years, Renée had respiratory issues, and this hounded her into her adult life. She never complained as she dismissed her illness nonchalantly—a behavioral trait in many nurses. Not one to share her innermost secrets, Renée was very private, and I respected that. Our paths collided some mornings at the end of her night shift and the beginning of my morning shift. I was happy to see her on those occasions, even though our visits were brief. At the end of her nursing shift, she is tired and ready for bed. Preparing to attend to my nursing caseload, I can only extend a quick nod, smile, or hug as I gush with pride. Personal and professional journeys unmistakably glued through blood and career. Because of her respiratory issues, Renée often overslept. When she did not turn up for her shift on time, it did not immediately set off any warning bells. However, after numerous calls and texts and after getting no response at the door, the apprehension escalated. Summoning the sheriff's department with anxiety and fear welling up in the bottom of my stomach was not easy. It was the beginning of a nightmare of what was to be the worst day of my life. It was a nightmare that changed our lives forever.

And so, it was that on February 15, 2014, as I was marking time by pacing in my living room, I heard a knock on my front door. When I opened the door, two officers from the Charlotte County Sheriff's department were male and a female. The female officer asked if I would like to sit down. I immediately knew this was not good news, and I knew then that life as I knew it was to be no more. I will remember the officer's words until the day that the last breath leaves my body. She said:

> *"I regret to inform you that your daughter Renée was found deceased."*

After numerous failed attempts to reach her, the Sheriff's department accessed her apartment. I remember slumping in the chair. The date of Renée's departure, tattooed on my brain forever, carved out a piece of me, and a part of me died.

I vaguely remember calling my sister Florence and my friend Irene. I called Alicia, her sister, who was living in Michigan at the time.

> *"There was no one at home with me at the time—no one was with me when I heard the news."*

However, in no time, family and friends came from near and far to offer support. In the next few days, it seemed as if I was never alone with this unbearable grief.

I drifted through the proceeding days in a bewildered state. Family and friends were always at my side, which was a blessing on one hand. On the other hand, I was merely existing, floating through life. I gave directions and followed instructions very well, as if I were in a surreal state of mind. It was as if I was transitioning into another life—another person—nothing was real—nothing made sense. She was deceased at home in her bed, which usually causes concern. An autopsy had to be completed by the authorities. They had to make sure there was no foul play, and it was not homicide. Having to wait until we had permission to conduct a funeral service without the final cause of death was ever so hard. Knowing and not knowing confounded the process even further.

We had to advise family members and friends living abroad of Renée's passing. We also had to advance the funeral service's date to give our loved ones time to obtain travel visas to attend the funeral. Her personal belongings had to be accessed and distributed to others. Notifications had to be placed in the media so that her friends would know about her passing and the date and time of the services. All the things we take for granted when it is someone else's experience were now our responsibility.

> *"I remember traveling to the celebration of life for my daughter. I wanted to scream from the pit of my stomach for someone to stop the madness and bring me back to reality."*

My mind raced during those days and even more so on the day of the funeral. "This situation was lunatic," I thought. I have two daughters—"where is Renée?" "Where are we going? This event is not real!" Children should outlive their parents. I had to bury my firstborn. In her tender years, and despite her respiratory condition, Renée had seen me struggling with a marriage destined for the court steps. Although she could not have understood everything at such a young age, my uncertainty and anxiety from the serious medical condition were not lost. Her quiet, reflective stance that I observed later in her life had an empathetic quality well beyond her years. She was the one who gave me purpose and a reason to keep rising stronger. Where the heck was my firstborn? How could this possibly be happening to her sister and me?

I remember how broken-hearted we all were when the usher started the tape with Andrea Bocelli's and Sarah Brightman's rendition of the song "Time to Say Goodbye." There was not a dry eye in the pews—each person reflecting on his or her recent or "not so recent" loss.

> *"The haunting yet comforting lyrics helped us to slowly rock and embrace the spirit of our loved ones: Renée; parents; friends' children, brothers, nieces, and nephews—family and friends— gone too soon and never to be forgotten."*

As we embraced the beautiful melody of love, praise, and freedom, I recalled my parents' unconditional love so many years ago.

> *"No matter what happened during our time together, the unconditional love that a mother shares with her children never diminishes—neither life events nor untimely death can ever separate me from that love."*

The lyrics, melancholy in its melodies, reminded me of the plans I had for our family—of the short time we experienced with this beautiful child—and the things I had to continue doing even though she was no longer here with us.

> *The finality of the word "goodbye" was a poignant reminder of what could have been—the essence of who we were as a family—and what we shared.*

Thank God for Renée's sister Alicia, who never left my side during those transitioning periods. As the firstborn, Renée helped to reshape my life and perspective when I experienced the darkness and personally imposed shame of a broken marriage. The daughter sent a knowing smile and produced indelible rays of sunshine during uncertain days. I remember the hollowness—the futility I experienced after I had processed the news that she was indeed gone—a void that still exists today.

> *"The pain, loss, and emptiness consume me year after year. Some days are better than others. My emotions fail me sometimes. Grief is not static. It does not end.*

Grief stings and pours salt into our wounds. I am consumed with sharp, overwhelming pain with no solace. I sometimes cry until my heart aches for the first child I held to my bosom as a gift from God. I cry until there are no more tears. Tears are like the gasoline you pour into an empty tank. When I am out of tears, there are no "tear-stations" to fill up. Those are the days when darkness engulfs me, and if I allow it to swallow me into a pit of doom, that is where I will remain. Other days, I can squeeze laughter from my belly and remember her life with happiness.

> *"The cruelest part of the tragedy is that the autopsy revealed that Renée died from a bad case of pneumonia. An illness easily fixed with a good dose of antibiotics. The very medicine that my daughter gives to her patients each day could have saved her life."*

I could rage against the unfairness of it all. What good would that do? How would I turn back the hands of the clock? I try to comfort myself that Renée is no longer suffering or in pain. It does not stop me from wishing she were here. I know that she would want me to continue living. That is what comforts me each day that I feel a melt-down coming. But it is tough! Working through my grief has been challenging. It was extremely difficult to talk about it at first.

> I "have tried to focus on the fact that "the show must go on." On whose terms? I am aware that each of us needs to contribute to society."

If we want better communities, we have to be intentional about creating initiatives that drive change. I cope with my grief by making a difference in someone's life. I focus on mentoring young people—helping them to devise a plan for their future. Whether I encounter them at work or in the community, I encourage them to aim higher. If they are open and receptive to my counsel, I urge them to go back to school and make higher education a priority. My sole objective is to engage them in positively essential conversations about advancement opportunities. The decision to accept or reject my counsel is up to them. Hopefully, long after our paths crossed, they will continue to water the seeds I planted.

Grief is processed differently by each individual. There are no "real" guidebooks when you are the recipient. My advice to others who encounter grief is to not impose a timeline on it. I say to them that no one can understand until they have experienced this kind of loss. Family and friends will say: "I understand" and "I know how you feel." The truth is no one indeed does. We all cope with grief in our own time—and there is no set time frame for when my grief will end. I did not receive formal grief counseling, though I conversed with friends who had similar experiences before Renée passed. Looking back, I think I should have explored that option, though it is not too late.

> *"I also find it therapeutic to continue some of the travel activities my children and I shared before Renée passed."*

I continue to frequently travel with family and friends and live my life to the fullest. "Longevity has its place" (Martin Luther King). King said the quality of life is more significant than the quantity. I have always maintained that waiting until retirement day to enjoy my life is ill-advised.

> *"My daughter Renée passed at age 35, long before traditional retirement age."*

There is still a lot of "what ifs" surrounding Renée's passing. We will never honestly know if anything could have prevented the date and time of her death. However, my advice to healthcare workers, who ignore their health, is not to take symptoms for granted. Research suggests that medical professionals build robust immune systems because of frequent exposure to sick patients. While this may be the long-term experience of some medical professionals, everyone's situation is different. Remember, regardless of research, every individual's immune system is unique. It is strongly dependent upon many factors: medical history, tenure in the medical environment, physical adaptability to new strains, and external conditions (e.g., pandemics). Like any other profession, heavy workloads may also prevent medical professionals from seeking medical attention. They may also self-diagnose—a second or third opinion is highly encouraged. As healthcare workers, we do not always have the answers. Take time to follow up on symptoms and get treated accordingly.

Through all the upheavals after losing Renée, I did not lose my faith in God. My faith in God has been a source of strength. I have a relationship with God. I see him as a friend who knows all my weaknesses and strengths. I know that I can always count on him. I reached out and continue to reach out daily to him for guidance, wisdom, and the power to go on.

> *"As painful and as unfair as it seems, I believe that God had Renée's purpose all worked out. You will recall that the doctor could not hear a heartbeat, and I had to have emergency surgery to save her life. God gave us a second chance then. I had her for thirty-six years later. He knew what he was doing. Now, it was her time to go. I am so grateful for thirty-six years!"*

I just do not believe I need organized religion to have that relationship. One of the bible scriptures I regularly read states, *"If I speak in the tongues of men and angels, but have not love, I am a nosy gong or a clanging cymbal"* (Corinthians 13:1). Today, I focus on my daughter Alicia and her family. I am grateful for our journey together. Naming her was no mistake. Alicia means *"noble natured."* I am also fortunate to be the proud grandmother of a beautiful grandson named Quentin. I try my *absolute best* to nurture and sustain a positive relationship with them. I am by no means a perfect human being or mother. I find delight in a favorite bible text:

> *"The Lord is my light and my salvation, whom shall I fear? The Lord is the stronghold of my life, of whom shall I be afraid?"*
> *(Psalm 27:1-2).*

Like any other person in life, I have my regrets—things I would do a lot differently if I had a do-over. I am working diligently not to leave any stones unturned as I continue to be the best person I can be—to live my best life. I am incredibly blessed to keep that in mind as I cherish the relationship with my daughter Alicia.

> *"Alicia has had to deal with the loss of her sister, trying to cope with her loss in her unique way. Together the both of us will get through, not over our loss."*

I admire Alicia's resilience and her desire to excel at whatever she pursues. Alicia studied and has flourished as a nurse. It is gratifying to see my daughter excel as a wife, mother, and caregiver. As her mother, I want her to know that I am incredibly proud of her. What I now know with much certainty is that life is uncertain. We do not know the hour, day, minute, second, or the year when we transition. For some of us, it will be sooner—for others, later. So, with that in mind, I plan to live life to the fullest, doing whatever good I can along the way.

> *"If I speak in the tongues of men or angels but do not have love, I am only a resounding gong or a clanging cymbal. If I have the gift of prophecy and can fathom all mysteries and all knowledge, and if I have faith that can move mountains but do not have love, I am nothing. If I give all I possess to the poor and give over my body to hardship that I may boast, but do not have love, I gain nothing"* (1 Corinthians 13:1-3)

Reflection Exercise
Renée' Story

If you are a parent grieving a child's loss, what lessons did you learn from Hyacinth's experience? How have you dealt with such a horrific loss? What will you do to work through your grief?

CHAPTER 7: CHRISTOPHER'S "GIFTS"

By
Beth *Marie* Wilson-Smalling
Aunt of
Christopher Craig-Anthony Taylor

Every day the media provides stories of accidents and horrible events that wipe out several family members at once. We hear about single and sometimes malicious events that take a child's life. We read about people being in the wrong place at the wrong time and who gets caught in crossfires—dragging them into a war they did not start. Recently, we heard about the horrific event of a caravan attack and nine family and friends killed during the crossfire. We also read about family members drowning when a barge sank to the bottom of the seas in California and wondered how these families cope after one incident changed the course of their lives forever.

No matter how many tragedies we read about or see on television, nothing prepares us for the news that our loved ones: a brother, his wife, two children, and his nephew were involved in a fatal car crash. The car was on the side of the road because of a flat tire. They had already replaced the tire and merged onto the highway. Of the five *people* traveling through Pennsylvania on their way to Washington, DC, to pursue an entrepreneurial venture, four of them were pronounced deceased. The father, and his two children, were pronounced dead at the scene. His nephew was airlifted to the hospital because the paramedics found a pulse. His physical injuries were so severe that the doctors could not do anything for him. Subsequently, Christopher's gifts saved the lives of others.

A recent television news report indicated that one organ donor could save seventy-five lives. While we want our loved ones with us, it is comforting to know that others benefited from this tragedy. People are alive because he died. Somewhere in the world, Christopher's heart beats; his lungs breathe, his kidneys are cleansing, and his liver is detoxifying. May the recipients deeply appreciate Christopher's "gifts."

The carnage, caused by a speeding eighteen-wheeler, drove over one section of the car, crushing the driver and his youngest son sitting immediately behind him. The driver's wife, an older son, and nephew were ejected from the vehicle and thrown several feet away. In one devastating event, four family members died because one person's action stopped them in their tracks and ravaged the dreams of an entire immediate and extended family.

Although I want to write about my big brother Horace and his children, Darren (15-years-old) and Shane (13-years-old), I will leave their personal story for another time. In this chapter, I want to focus on my nephew Christopher Craig-Anthony Taylor, a vibrant 17-year-old who had experienced more than his fair share of challenges and who was on the right track when he passed.

On December 20, 1985, Christopher was born in Kingston, Jamaica, to my sister Diane Wilson-Carter and Donavon Taylor. It was a challenging period in Diane's life because the relationship ended long before the child was born. His father was not available, and Diane pretty much went through the pregnancy by herself and with the support of her family. As her older sister, being the protective type, I made myself available to take her to her various appointments and be there for Christopher's birth.

It was a fascinated experience because, at that time, I did not have any children. I was learning about the process through my sister's eyes. While it was not a difficult birth, he was not a small baby. His personality was as large as his physical weight and height. He was an effervescent child. It was evident to everyone who came in contact with him that he would be a strong force of nature. Diane and Christopher were remarkably close. He was her world, and she doted on him. For the first three years of Christopher's life, Diane shared a house with our oldest brother Horace and his wife. As a result, Christopher looked up to Horace as a male parent, and the surrogate parental bond was powerful.

About three years after Christopher was born, Diane met and fell in love with her husband, Norman—a fine gentleman she met through her friend and colleague at work. At the time, Norman was living in New York City. They were a devoted couple and the envy of everyone in their circles. Diane had her second child, the first child with Norman, in 1991 and migrated to the United States a few years later. She, hearing of the hardship of living in a new country with young children, was persuaded to leave the children in Jamaica with her mother. This strategy allowed the affectionate couple to get settled into their new home. The children joined their parents in New York City a couple of years later (the mid-1990s), making Christopher about 9-10-years-old.

Christopher and his sister Christine's adjustment were challenging—a new blended family, country, culture, home, school system, to name a few. Neither child had lived with their parents consistently, and this caused some uneasiness in the home dynamics. At about 13-years-old, during puberty, he adopted a more rebellious persona. Through no fault of his parents, changing family dynamics can be complicated for everyone, like any blended family. Christopher sought friendships with others who had opposing values than his parents and family. Research shows that kids reach puberty at around age 13 to 14. Most parents and teachers believe that rebellion at puberty is against them. On the contrary, researchers believe the insurgency is not against parents—it is only acted against them (Pickhardt, 2009).

> *"Children are trying to shed their persona under parental control to find their own identity. It is not uncommon for them to explore various options."*

Naturally, Christopher preferred to "hang" with his friends on basketball courts and elsewhere—anywhere but home. To appease his challenges and escape the rules at home, he stayed out late, avoided his chores, and became argumentative with his parents.

Christopher ran away from home for several days because he refused to conform to the house rules. During his constant association with the wrong crowd, he was accused of petty theft by an associate. As a result, he was detained in a New York Juvenile Detention facility for a few months, only to have the case dismissed by the court. Upon rejecting the claim and subsequent dismissal of the case, Christopher saw this as an opportunity to change the course of his life. He chose to live with his uncle,

Horace, and his family. His cousins had a positive influence on his life, and in no time, the family observed a positive difference in his appearance, outlook, choices, and decisions.

He attended church regularly with the family, returned to high school, and did very well. He also became involved in the youth group at church. After six months of living with our brother Horace, Diane was thrilled with Christopher's progress. You will recall that Horace had been in Christopher's life within the first three years of his birth. Bonds formed early in a child's life are vital and impermeable. At one point, he called Horace "Daddy." The paternal connection with Horace was more potent than any other. Like everyone in the family, I was relieved that there was a light at the end of the tunnel. Christopher was determined to take charge of his life by turning things around. He was safe from the perils of the street—and he was given much credit for trying.

Imagine our anguish when Horace and the three boys died soon after. On Friday, July 18, 2003, around 9:00 a.m., I worked on my sister Diane's resume and called her to discuss it. When I called her direct line, a strange voice answered the phone. Upon confirming my relationship with Diane, the lady told me to call my aunt. Diane had left work due to a family emergency. Our mother was living with Diane, and I thought that the crisis was with her. When I called my aunt, she explained that Horace had died in a car accident. There was no other report about anyone else. I called my younger brother, Dean instructing him to call Diane's husband, Norman, for details. By the time I got to Dean's house, I had heard that our brother Horace, and his children, Darren, and Shane, had also passed. Reportedly, Rhona, Horace's wife, and Christopher were in the hospital.

My brother Dean and I made the road trip to Pennsylvania to visit Christopher and Rhona at the hospital. We received updates from the family and connected in every way we could. The family came from far and wide to converge at the hospital. Christopher was on life support with severe brain and other internal injuries. The doctors could do nothing else for him. The chaplain came and prayed with the family before the doctors took him to the operating room to harvest his transferable organs.

Christopher's sister, Christine, had a dream where she was conversing with her brother. He told her that he died in the "chopper" that airlifted him to the hospital. He also said that he had an out-of-body experience floating above and looking at himself on the bed. He was able to name and describe everyone who was in that room and where they stood. He did not have the Chaplin's name — the person described as the strange black man who prayed. Christine had refused to see her brother in that condition. Although she did not enter his hospital room, she could describe the room in detail based on her conversation in her dream with her brother. Assured that her brother had made peace with his situation, she felt at ease.

Horace's wife, Rhona, was the only one who physically survived the accident. She spent less than one week in the hospital. My sister-in-law could not go home for months.

> *"Understandably, she was in a daze for years, even now questioning her right to be happy—sixteen years after the tragedy."*

The funeral services were delayed because of police investigations. Burying four family members at once was painfully overwhelming for the family. I do not know how we managed to keep it together. The decision to cremate Christopher's body and lay his remains in Valhalla, New York, was a welcomed one.

I was devastated and unable to understand why something like this could have happened. My children were confused about the loss of their uncle and three first cousins. I questioned the reality of it. It did not seem real. Time stood still. At the time of the tragedy, I lived in Georgia. While I regularly spoke with my family, I had not seen them since the spring of that year. Horace's multilevel marketing business was doing well. He was traveling to Maryland to attend a conference where he would receive an award. He decided to take his family with him as a mini vacation. The summer before, Horace's two boys joined us in Georgia for vacation. The boys were doing very well academically, and they were such good souls. During this challenging time, a conversation with God is fraught with confusion.

From my perspective, grieving comes and goes because of the physical distance. My brother and his family lived in New York, and I lived in Georgia. I did not see them daily or even monthly. However, we spoke on the telephone regularly and visited each other's homes at least once per year. I sometimes think about needing to call my brother Horace about a joke or with some snippet of news.

> *"The family pictures moved on without Horace and my nephews. I miss Horace because I am unable to shoot the breeze with him on his birthday and special holidays."*

On occasions when something funny happens in my life, I want to share the joke with him. While my faith remains strong, I often have moments when I take a ride into a world of visualization and regret.

Our family lost one man and three male children that morning. This year Horace would have been 65, Darren

32, Shane 30, and Christopher 35 years of age. I would imagine that if they had lived, our family would be significantly larger by now. Assuming the three boys would select a spouse and have children of their own, our family tree would have many more branches. My brother's legacy lives on in his two older children from a previous marriage: Damien and Deanne. Horace would have been happy to know that Damien now has four children. I imagine that Horace would continue to be a phenomenal son, spouse, father, brother, grandfather, and friend. I pray that we will meet again someday. In his passing, my sister's son Christopher, my nephew, my mother's grandson, my children's cousin lives on in others:

> *"Through organ donation, other ligaments, and tissues, Christopher contributed greatly to medical research."*

"Now faith is the substance of things hoped for, the evidence of things not seen" (Hebrews 11:1: KJV). I pray I will see them again some sweet day. Keep the faith and keep Rising Stronger™.

> *"Jesus looked at them and said, "With man this is impossible, but with God, all things are possible." (Matthew 19:26)*

CHAPTER 8: URBAN ATROCITIES

By
Ingrid Anonymous
Mother of
Dennis and Zack Anonymous

I was born in a rural town in one of the fourteen parishes of Jamaica. I migrated to Kingston, the fast-paced megapolis capital of Jamaica, at an early age. Deep down, I was a country girl at heart. Even today, people from Kingston never fail to remind migrants of their birthplace and origin. I lived with one of my aunts, a sister to my mother. My grandfather was a white gentleman with blond hair and green eyes. He was more than six feet tall, and to a young impressionable child, he and other family members appeared like giants. His wife, my grandmother, was a dark-skinned woman of profound African heritage and deep brown eyes. My grandparents had eight children, one of whom was my mother. So, it was not surprising that our complexion, culture, and heritage collided with Scottish and African origins. Although outsiders questioned our light skin-tone, those who lived in the village knew its roots. Both my parents were from Jamaica and lived in the "country" (rural areas). Although I spent most of the year with my aunt in Kingston, I returned to the country for holidays with my parents. These visits provided just enough time to bond with my family but not enough time to get to know the community or the village where I was born.

In the late 1960s, I met and fell in love with a genuinely nice young man in Kingston, Jamaica. At the time, I had no idea who he was or what he did. In my naiveté, I did not even know how popular he was. He had dark skin like my grandmother and the whitest set of ivory teeth that you could see a mile off. He was attractive, wildly charming, and was enough to sweep me off my feet. To this day, he can open my heart and light my life. I still blush just thinking about some of our peculiar antics in the early days. Everyone who saw us together knew we were in love. Heck, we knew we were a match for each other, and we could go places.

Five years after we became an exclusive couple, our first child, a boy, was born. We were ecstatic and giddy with happiness. Naturally, the boy had both our features, cementing the diversity of cultures that started with my grandparent's union. The second child was born in 1977, and yes—it was a girl. We did not realize that she would be the only girl we would have of our four children. Nine years after we met, we formalized our union, and we became man and wife.

Our third child, alias Dennis, was born in the late 1980s. Dennis, a healthy baby, was in a hurry to be born and screamed his way into the world. He started crying before he fully emerged from my womb. Once Dennis knew it was time to emerge from the protection of the womb, Dennis was ready to face the world. He pushed his way into the world with enthusiasm and urgency. The baby had beautiful hazel eyes and noticeably lighted brown skin. He was born with a peculiar blonde hair texture that was nerve-racking. He came with everything that his mixed Scottish and African ancestry had to offer. His original blond hair turned black at some point. He shared both our features—a fusion formed in love and manifesting in a giant-sized, compassionately expressive child.

Research suggests that babies who have developed physical and emotional faculties allow them to express imminent danger or painful stimuli. Long before Dennis reached age two, we learned that Dennis did not like to be confined—sequestering spaces were not his liking. He was a busy child—always extremely active. He drew people to him like a magnet. I remember a peculiar scenario about Dennis. As a toddler, he hated to be placed in his crib and left alone. After bathing him and setting him down for a nap, Dennis would somehow find himself outside of his crib, dragging his blanket behind him with a broad sheepish grin on his face. Each time we put him in the crib, he would find his way out.

> *"We decided to observe him see how he exited the crib. He lifted the mattress. One by one, he set the crib boards aside and stepped out of the crib from the bottom. No need to climb from the top. He slid easily through the bottom."*

He did not like being tethered—he preferred his freedom. To escape his playpen, he would bounce it over and around, stepping out of it as if he was a grown man. It seemed like Dennis grew up without us knowing it—he was a big boy. Despite his exploits, he was a smart, vibrant child who gave us no problems.

His adventures, however, frightened us. I am still trying to figure out how a 9-year-old boy could learn to drive an adult car. Plato's theory that knowledge is innate rings real today as I reflect on Dennis's progression. I was in the house one day when I glanced up to see the reflection of my car. Mesmerized and uncertain of what was happening, I watched the shadows of the vehicle against the window curtains. Try as I might, I could not see who was sitting in the driver's seat as the car slowly moved below the window. When I ran outside to see what was happening, my 9-year-old son, Dennis, intentionally drove the car out of the sun. I did not know whether to laugh or cry. I kept a close eye on my car keys from then on. Dennis was about ten years old and still in prep school when, upon observing the road being tarred and paved, he was burned accidentally by the hose filled with hot burning tar. His leg, more so than his hands and face, were burned, yet he was able to overcome those challenges. He was a curious child who did not always pay attention to his environment. A motorist hit him on the way home from school one day. Much to our relief, the damage was minimal.

One tussle with his older brother led to a concussion that took us to the hospital in Kingston. It was certainly not something to laugh about as it was terrifying. He was thrown to the ground to prove a point, where he accidentally hit his head, giving him a concussion. We were beside ourselves with anxiety as we rushed him to the hospital. He survived that escapade to tell the story over and over. One evening, he took his father's car to visit his girlfriend. He was fourteen or fifteen years old. He took the car without our knowledge. Upon his return, supposedly a crazy driver racing down the road crashed into the back of the car just as he turned into our driveway. The vehicle was entirely wrecked, and Dennis ran frantically inside to tell his brothers what had happened. Our feelings were mixed. Anger and happiness are two of the emotions that come to mind at the moment.

Early in life, Dennis picked up cues on dress code, grooming, and appearance from his father, known for his fashionable attire. Besides, his father was always attending important meetings, so formal attire was essential. Like his dad, Dennis loved cologne—it was considered a *chick magnet* to look and smell good. Dennis was always getting into a pickle with his siblings since he liked to get into their things when he was splashed carelessly on every inch of his body. The running joke was that Dennis's older brother would lock his room door to preserve his expensive cologne. Dennis would jimmy the lock so that he could get into his brother's room to use his cologne. His brother caught him after setting a trap for him one day. The two boys could not help but get into a brawl over Dennis's cleverness. The family still laughs about that incident. Dennis was fearlessly adventurous.

When he was older, we allowed Dennis to apprentice at a mechanic shop in Kingston, Jamaica. His passion for fixing things with his hands had started to spread in our circles. He was able to analyze and diagnose mechanical problems that were troublesome for others. He did not take long to figure things out either. Despite his desire to go directly into that career, the cultural consensus was that he needed to stay in school for a traditional high school diploma. Although Dennis preferred working with his hands, he passed his high school examination and went to various liberal arts high schools—indeed not his first choice.

Dennis's male friends loved hanging out with him because he could attract many ladies to the clubs they visited. His charismatic personality and effortless approach to people opened many doors for him. His friends always joked about being able to benefit from the overflow of ladies who flocked him. As a result of his engaging, adventurous personality, our house had many visitors. Everyone wanted to be around him. As the chief entertainer in the household, he provided food and drinks for everyone.

Even though Dennis was the third child, he was the first child to leave home. He was in a hurry to see the world and to explore all that it had to offer. Dennis arrived in the United States late 1990s. We had our United States residency for several years and waited until the children completed high school before making the formal move. He was excited about a mechanical engineering career. Since we were not yet ready to make the final move, Dennis joined a friend's family, where he stayed for a while. Already, there was trouble in the household. My friend had asked her son to leave home as he was violating the rules of the house. Dennis, the mediator that he was, would cover for the son of my friend. He was always approached with suspicion and skepticism by my friend. She did not know where extra male clothing was coming from and believed he was sneaking strangers into her home. Due to the fallout, he did not get to go to mechanic school as promised. Dennis was trying to help her son, who was secretly visiting the home, to wash his clothes and get something to eat when she was not present. My son was an unrepentant enabler. *His mantra was: "Everyone deserves a second chance."* The environment had become controversial, and he had to leave my friend's house.

Dennis rented an apartment and worked one or two jobs to meet his expenses. We met his requests for extra cash and supported him as best as we could. Subsequently, he decided it was too much to keep asking us for supplementary income. He felt guilty and tried to fix the situation by himself. He did not fully comprehend the American culture and, as a result, made some colossal mistakes in managing the bills. Much to my chagrin, Dennis was evicted from his apartment and was unable to retrieve much of his belongings. Not being there when the eviction occurred, spectators took what they could physically carry with them. He had made friends with a young lady in the apartment complex and afterward moved in at her invitation. The relationship blossomed, and they later had a beautiful daughter.

I brought my youngest son, Zach, to the United States to visit his brother at the turn of the new century. Zach wanted to attend university. Despite the 2-year separation, both boys bonded well. They were closer in age than the older siblings, and they balanced each other well. The plan was to get both boys an apartment and return to Jamaica. I helped Dennis to rebuild his credit by paying off his bills. I stayed with the boys for about 1-2 months and then decided to stay and help them settle in. My husband, their father, was still in Jamaica, so the intention was to help the boys settle in and then return home.

Dennis did not discriminate when choosing friends. He had compassion for the underdog. My son identified the good in everyone and was always willing to accept people who had gone through struggles and were fighting their way back to the surface—endeavoring to rise stronger. He met Jason, a young man who moved to his town supposedly away from a lifestyle of poor choices. Jason wanted a better life, and the city offered a compelling argument—much better than his previous city. Career and family prospects were essential to both young men.

Dennis and his friend Jason celebrated their birthdays within days of each other. Dennis was working on his birthday, so he did not get to celebrate with his friends. A week before Jason's birthday, he called Dennis to invite him to a club to celebrate both birthdays.

That very same Saturday, I tiptoed by Dennis's workplace. I was tired after a long day standing at work. I knew that seeing him would be an exciting, gregarious experience—one that would entail being lifted off the ground and spun around several times. Much as I love my enthusiastic son, I was too tired for the hassle that day and sneaked quietly by the mechanic shop, hoping to avoid him that day. He could not help himself. It was as if he could sense that I was there. The minute he saw me across the street, he ran out and hugged me tightly. He gave me some kisses on my face as he was so excited to see me. I asked him why he was wearing a cap, and he said because his hair needed cutting. He is usually well-groomed, so I was surprised that he had allowed the hair to grow bushy and unkempt.

> *"He assured me that next time I saw him, his hair would be groomed. That was the last time I saw him alive."*

Even though I was tired and tried to avoid him, that hug and those kisses were the last time my son held me. Hindsight is always 20/20. We know not the day or the hour when our lives will turn upside down and around. I wish I were not as tired on that last day. I long for the days when my son wrapped me with the strong arms of his tall Scottish great-grandpapa, spinning my slender frame round and round. I long for the times when he was the center of attention, and his friends would sit around him, hanging on to his every word.

> *"Dennis was murdered several weeks after his only daughter was born. No, he did not die in a true sense. His life was snuffed out of him—plucked out by a vicious, coldhearted individual whose identity is as cold as the act itself."*

The following day I returned from work to see many people in my apartment, including my last son Zach. Zach said, *"Dennis dead—dem kill him."* That is all I remembered as I dropped my bag and ran out to the street in a mad frenzy. I do not know how they caught me or where they caught me. All I know is that I had to find my son.

> *"He told me I would see him again with his haircut. He was 21 years of age. Where was he? Lord, have mercy!"*

Dennis's favorite color was blue. No, it is not the cliché—*blue is for boys*. He naturally loved blue as a boy and as a man—some men like black, white, green, or red. My son loved blue. Dennis's girlfriend said that he went to Walmart the day before, and he bought blue decorative accessories for the bathroom. He was stylish, and his apartment was reflective of that style. He was the one who loved to clean and keep an orderly apartment. When his girlfriend returned from work that morning, she had a refurbished bathroom. Her mother said that Jason, his friend, came to wake him up. He got out of his bed, where he was sleeping with the baby in the room. Dennis gave his girlfriend's mother the baby. He instructed her to look after her because he was going out with Jason. There were times when Dennis stayed at my home if he was out too late and he was closer to my apartment.

> *"Dennis did not return home that night, and he was not with me. His girlfriend was distraught that he had not come home."*

Jason was driving his girlfriend's car, and she, too, was concerned. Never in a million years would anyone suspect that someone killed both men the night before. They wanted to avoid a busy, congested highway and decided to take the backroads as many people do in some cities.

Allegedly, someone killed them on those backroads. The assailant(s) took their wallets with all their contents and shot them. Dennis must have put his hands up to protect his face as he had one bullet in his hand. Reportedly, one of the shots came from Jason and entered Dennis. The car crashed into a ditch, and the assailant(s) disappeared into thin air: multiple stories and speculations circulated about what happened that night.

Because Dennis's death was a homicide, I did not know where to send his body. I had been living here only a few short months. I was a grieving mother in a strange land. Someone suggested that we send it to a small boutique funeral home. It was much farther away from where we lived. I could not bring myself to go to the funeral home before the funeral. Besides, I did not have a car to get around.

> *"We were practicing Catholics, so his father, who lived in Jamaica, came up and made final arrangements."*

On Dennis's memorial day, the church had many patrons of the mechanic shop where he worked. As young as my son was, he was well-known and respected in the community. His family came from Jamaica and elsewhere, and we laid him to rest. We later had a memorial service in Jamaica to allow our local family and friends to mourn our loss. People came from near and far to celebrate his life.

The murder of my son and his friend Jason remains cold cases. No one has been formally arrested and charged with their murders. The police never found the murder weapons.

> *"All I know is that my third child is never coming home again. His daughter did not get to see him beyond her few weeks on earth— not enough time to bond—to get to know each other."*

His daughter has had to grow up without her father. She had no choice—someone stole that option from her. She graduated high school a short while ago, and I am sure that she needs answers like us. Sometimes I feel as if I took my child like a lamb to the slaughter. His family, siblings, and I lost so much. Our lives will never be the same. Our burdens are enormous, and our sacrifices are even more immense.

> *"Losing a child is a horrific experience that no parent should bear. Losing a child at the hands of another is even more painful."*

Grief stings like the gill of a pelican swooping into the sea to feast on the spoils and then souring triumphantly into the air. In retrospect, I wish I sought grief counseling. I closed my heart and inhaled the pain each day. My husband sought counseling in Jamaica. In the ensuing months, I memorized our last encounter. I remembered the times before when Dennis squeezed me with his strong arms as he embraced me. We will always painfully remember that Dennis is dead at the hands of a monster. We may never know who, what, or why. We will never forget Dennis. Our lives will never be the same.

Dennis's murder was only the first of two horrendous nightmares with our family. His younger brother, Zach, an academically astute young man who had served in the United States military, was also murdered years later. You will recall that our youngest child Zach accompanied me to the United States to attend college. However, after his brother died, Zach enlisted in the United States military. Like many soldiers, he faced numerous challenges.

> *"The awful, tragic, and blood-curdling pain returned. This time our baby boy is gone. It is as if we are reliving Dennis's passing once again. The wound is too raw to discuss at this time."*

Just as we thought that we were managing the grief of losing one child, we had to start grieving for another child. Our burdens are enormous, and our sacrifices are considerable. Our hearts remain broken over the loss of the three young men in this story.

> *"He who dwells in the shelter of the most High will rest in the shadow of the almighty. I will say of the Lord, "He is my refuge and my fortress, my God, in whom I trust." Surely he will save you from the fowler's snare and from the deadly pestilence" (Psalm 91: 1-3: NIV)*

The pain will never go away. However, our faith is here to stay. Faith keeps us strong and helps us to manage our grief. The monsters who killed our children have no hold on our hearts. Our hearts scream love for our four children. Martin Luther King declares:

> *"Darkness cannot drive out darkness; only love can do that. Hate cannot drive out hate; only love can do that."*

Thank you for keeping our family in your prayers. We will not lose heart! Through our unwavering faith, we will keep Rising Stronger™!

What can you do to manage the grief that you or a loved one is experiencing today?

CHAPTER 9: DEADLY INTENTIONS

By
Sharon A White-Answer Carter
Mother of
Georgia A. Green-Lee

Red was my daughter's favorite color. Before I get into the tragedy of her passing, let me get that one emotional yet straightforward fact out into the universe. It has been forty and a half years since I had my first child. I remember that day as if it were yesterday. Georgia was the first of my two daughters. On Thursday, July 5, 1979, she came into my life at 2:20 p.m., weighing 7.5 pounds. I was an immature young girl, shy of sixteen-years-old. I did not even realize I was pregnant until I was four months along. That may have been a good thing—the first four months of my pregnancy were stress-free. By the time word got around at school that I was pregnant, I was almost ready to give birth. Although my parents were not happy with the situation, I had their loving support. The baby was born during the summer months, so my high school education was uninterrupted.

I was fortunate to be in a school system that encouraged young mothers to continue with their education. The guidance counselor at my high school referred me to a new program designed for teenaged mothers. By joining the program, I would be allowed to complete any gaps in my high school education. Since my baby was the first grandchild for both families, everyone played indispensable roles. The family members of Georgia's father were supportive. His older sister, Sonya, took me to all my prenatal visits and accompanied me to register for the program designed for teens. There, I gained access to counseling and other resources.

Georgia's birth was not difficult, despite the stress and anxiety when I found out I was pregnant. I had less than six months to prepare for her entrance into the world. Tapping into the resources available to me was not hard. She made her entrance as if she were here before, clinging onto me with a powerful grip. Like a baby craving for compassion and love, her warm, tender body laid claim to my comfortable bosom and a huge heart. She was ready to make up for the time I was not aware of her presence. While I was in the recovery room with two other mothers, the nurse walked right by me, looking for her mother. I recalled saying to the nurse in a small voice, *"She is mine. She is mine."* My voice became increasingly higher and my confidence stronger as I accepted the role in this child's life—mother, mama, mom, mommy. I claimed her as she had claimed me. The nurse asked, *"How do you know she is yours when there are two other mothers in the room?"* I told her I knew she was mine because everything she was wearing, including the pins holding her cloth diaper, was blue. Though several cultures link blue to baby boys, the color, coupled with strength and stability, also symbolizes faith, allegiance, prudence, and self-confidence. I wanted her to grow into her destiny. The nurse hesitated before giving me, my daughter. I was a young, petite mother who was shy of sixteen years old. I weighed 120 pounds, with 62 inches in height. I prayed that the energy she emanated on that faithful morning would follow her throughout life.

Naturally, because I was so young and Georgia was my first child, the nurse was uncertain about my ability to hold and breastfeed her. She was exceedingly kind and supportive as she gently eased Georgia into my arms while providing instructions about these matters. I took my daughter to my bosom with the nurse observing me and winced as she snatched my breast with her hungry, determined lips. I recall an absence of fear and a bond that only babies, nurtured in the womb by their mother, can recognize. She clung on as if her life depended on it. She knew me, and I knew her. Despite my age and birth circumstances, I was determined to be the best mother to my daughter. I promised to follow God's guidance and be her provider and protector.

Despite being given a clean bill of health after Georgia was born, I was kept in the hospital for a couple of days due to my age. I returned home to my mother, who showed me how to take care of my baby. Two weeks after she was born, I sat my final annual school exam. While I was in school, Georgia spent time at the newly formed women's center and nursery, a few miles from where I attended high school. As one of the first babies in the program, she stamped her personality and precociousness on all the caregivers' hearts. Even forty years later, a couple of the remaining caregivers speak highly of my daughter. I doubt they knew her real name as she was so "grown-up" and independent that everyone called my baby girl "Ms. Rossie."

Georgia attended Kindergarten at age three and became involved in many extra-curricular activities, including her two favorites: swimming and dancing. She also enjoyed doing nails and later studied to be a nail technician. Georgia enjoyed people and socialized on every opportunity. I was very much involved in Georgia's life when she was growing up. I had to meet and vet her friends to ensure wise choices. She was eleven years old when she rescued one of her classmates, Nyocca, from playground bullies. She brought her home to introduce her to me, and over time, they declared themselves as 'sisters' and best friends for life.

Nyocca's mother and I became close friends. As teenage mothers, we had so much in common, and besides, the girls were inseparable. Georgia adopted Nyocca's brother as her brother too. She was that type of child—she hated injustice and unfairness. She was both a fierce protector of others and a defender against trespassers. As a young mother, it was easy for me to relate to my daughter's friends. Their parents welcomed my presence in their lives. With my organizational skills, social network, and flair for fashion and excitement, life with Georgia was good. I accompanied Georgia and her friends to social events to keep my promises to my daughter. When she showed interest in a boy, I shared my expectations for my daughter with him.

Georgia migrated to Florida at the age of eighteen and immersed herself in retail and childcare activities. She later entered into the consumer goods industry in various aspects of customer service. With her vibrant personality, customer service was spontaneous, and everyone loved her. Funny how children unknowingly declare their future. At age twelve, she professed she would marry young and have two children. She never wavered from that plan and made it known everywhere she went. It was a declaration she made to her family, close friends, intended or betrothed.

"Whether by coincidence or purpose, circumstances often collide into unexpected actions. I was not surprised when Georgia met and got married to Trevor A. Lee on January 23, 2000, nearly twenty years ago." Although I was not yet forty, I was over the moon when Trevor and Georgia had their first child. To my delight, I was solely responsible for naming my first grandchild.

> *"I was given an African book of names and meaning thirty-four years ago. In the book, the name Najja means "strong one"—"protector"—and "born after."*

It was my unconscious attempt to align my grandson with his generational position and, in some cases, refer to his brilliant, beautiful eyes. He had the vibrant, gregarious, and protective personality of his mother and his father's sturdy frame. He was a bright pink baby with a cute set of dimples and a broad, curious smile. His wit has not lost its luster, and I loved cuddling and squeezing his chubby face. He looked a lot like his father though I could see his mother's genes competing for attention.

At best, Trevor and Georgia were an outgoing couple with lots of friends. The first couple of years of their marriage were happy ones. I admired Georgia's strength and tenacity as a wife and mother. Although the marriage lost its sheen and things changed dramatically, Georgia held on to her childhood plan of having two children for the same man. She insisted that she would have a second child with Trevor. No one could talk her out of it—not even me. Five years later, Trevor and Georgia fulfilled their promises of having two children together. Beautiful baby girl Nia was born. Nia was the first girl in the blended family.

> *Nia is a Swahili name I found in the African book of names. The name has significance in the African American community—the fifth day of Kwanzaa, an African American celebration of life, which begins December 26 and ends January 1.*

It emphasizes creating a purpose-driven life for ourselves and our community. Quick online research indicates that Nia means aim, purpose, resolve, brilliance, vigor, and significance.

When Georgia and her sister were children, I taught them by example. I did not send them to church. I took them to church. I did not tell them to be kind and to give to others. I showed them how to be kind by being kind-hearted. Naturally, as children expand their social networks, they ultimately carve their paths and personalize their values. They create their own unique identity as they rebel or seek independence from their parents. Following my family's Christian values, Georgia instilled a strong sense of safety and stability for her family and did whatever she could to sustain those values in the home. She took Najja and Nia to church every Sunday morning.

You will recollect that when Georgia was born, I chose blue as her first color. I thought it blended better with her beautiful dark skin. At age nine, she declared that red was her favorite color, and I conformed to that request by ensuring she wore red all the time. As an adult, she maintained her personal color choice. This choice was symbolic of her birth month and a replica of her bold, extroverted, and passionate personality. Her house décor was black and white, and those who knew her well spoke highly of her propensity to entertain—a family trait she picked up from me.

"Georgia also had a knack for bringing family members together, despite objections to the contrary. For me, "once bitten, twice shy." Usually, I do not allow second and third chances. My daughter, on the other hand, forgives and forgets the minute she gives you a piece of her mind."

The family unit meant more to Georgia than parentage. She married into a somewhat blended family as Trevor had children before the marriage. She frequently opened her heart and their home to Trevor's older children. Georgia was an advocate, liaison, and mediator for them, helping to meet their emotional and financial needs. She wanted to ensure the siblings developed an impermeable bond without any rivalry. Even after her marriage to Trevor ended, she tried to keep the line of communication open. The three boys loved her, and they continue to speak openly of their affection for her.

On January 20, 2008, I was at home in Boston when I got the call that my daughter Georgia was shot and killed at 4:50 a.m. in Lauderhill, Florida, where she resided with her children. I was with my 17-year-old stepson while my fiancé was at work when I got the news.

> *"I was in a state of disbelief. I asked her brother: "Where is she? Is she breathing? Where is the (known perpetrator)? Where are my grandchildren? Have you called the police?"*

Her brother answered all the questions in a monotone voice. He was apparently in a fog. He told me that the police were "on the way." I told him to hang up and wait for their arrival. I immediately called my fiancé and then placed a call to my friend who lived in the apartment across from Georgia's apartment complex. I asked her to visit my daughter's apartment to see what was happening.

In my haziness, I recalled that two weeks before this devastating event, Georgia told me she had a dream that something terrible happened, and I was crying. In the dream, the rain was falling. There was someone in the back of a police car, and there was yellow tape. The images my friend described to me when she returned from my daughter's apartment were eerily similar to how Georgia had portrayed the scene in her dream. In reality, the person in the back of the police car was Georgia's brother and by no means the shooter. I asked my friend to take the telephone to one of the crime scene investigators to explain my relationship to Georgia and share what her brother had told me. It was at that point the officer said to me that my daughter was dead.

I could not stay on the phone with the police officer as my heart was throbbing way too fast. I was stunned and numb all at once. I laid on the floor for quite a while until my fiancée got home and picked me up about an hour later. I texted all my friends and family in my address book about Georgia's untimely passing. Georgia was the first baby in my inner sphere of influence. I could not bear for family and friends to hear the news on the radio or see it on television. The message had to come from me. As you can imagine, the phone kept ringing off the hook. Grief struck me like a ton of bricks. I was inconsolable and could not speak to anyone though I could indeed feel their prayers.

My fiancé immediately made plans for me to go to Florida the following day. I had already spoken to Trevor, Georgia's ex-husband, and the children's father. By now, he was living in Atlanta, Georgia, USA, and he was already on his way to Florida to get the children. The children went into protective custody immediately, a seemingly hazardous situation. A close family member needed to get there fast.

> *"Trevor spoke to Georgia only the Thursday before, and he too was stunned by the turn of events. Georgia's sister Jeniel spoke to her the night before she died."*

Plans were already in the works to travel from Jamaica to visit her sister the next day. When she got the news of her sister's death, she kept her travel plans, arriving that afternoon in time to visit with the children and their father. Their godmother, Nyocca, who lives in Florida, was also there.

I remember checking in for my flight at the airport when the agent commented on my Florida vacation plans. It was the middle of January, and here I was going to Florida. Indeed, it was to get away from the cold weather—right? I told her it was not a pleasant trip. I was going to bury my daughter—my first child. I think somehow saying those words were my tipping point.

> *"I lost all sense of control, and tears flowed like a river. I did not think I would ever stop crying. The lady came from behind the ticketing counter to console me. She patiently waited for me to gain composure."*

She booked me into first class—a blessing because I could not stop crying. Curled up in the fetal position in that huge seat, I was able to turn my eyes away from curious passengers as I "turned the tap on."

One of my friends picked me up at the airport and took me to her home. From then on, everything turned into a media sensation, legal investigations, and chase for the accused. For us, it was an overall emotional frenzy. My grandson Najja, the older of the two children, was visibly shaken. He was inconsolable. Counselors were on hand for the children, and more importantly, Trevor, Jeniel, and Nyocca comforted them. It was a vicious crime against the mother of two young children. People were horrified and empathetic all at once. Everyone, including the media, wanted the inside scoop. There were too many reporters waiting at the apartment, and I was not ready to speak publicly.

I went to the police station to speak with the detective in charge of the case. I had to get the necessary paperwork to start funeral arrangements. My "get it done" self-preservation personality kicked into high gear. Only when I paused for air could I feel the overwhelming assault and the flood of doom enveloping my spirit. Our family is blessed to have a local community of friends in Florida who stepped forward to do whatever they could to make the situation smoother. Other friends came from New York, England, Canada, and Jamaica to walk me through the funeral preparation process. I finally visited the apartment complex a couple of days later and spoke with some people there.

> *"The worst part of the experience was seeing my daughter and grandchildren's pictures all over the news. Losing a child is devastating—the pain triples when a deadly force causes that child's life."*

It is even worst when it is a known party to the deceased, children, and family. "How could you...........?" I felt like I was watching an episode of NCIS on American television. It did not feel like my life. I felt like I was taking a *sneak peek* into someone else's life. I do not think I felt anger at that moment. I was still locked in disbelief and operating in a trance-like state. Unfortunately, I was looking into the unfortunate outcome of my daughter's life. Our family dreams shattered. Saying that our family, friends, and confidants were shocked is, to put it mildly. We were thrown into this mayhem, whether we liked it or not. I was relieved after authorities finally caught the killer and put him behind bars.

As her mother, I was allowed to view her in the casket first. The funeral directors were kind enough to place a chair nearby for me to sit. My friend selected a lovely white dress for her. I put my hand on the beautiful dress and touched her lifeless face, void of her infectious smile and laughter. It was at that point that it hit me like a ton of bricks—this is it. I will never see her smiling face or never hear her laughter again. We will never have another *fight* about me moving to Boston and getting "*fat.*" Believe me that my move to Boston was a source of emotional contention coupled with an intense, aggressive fight between my daughter and me. She encouraged the relationship with my then-boyfriend because she admitted we were great together.

> ["You no fraid "dem tief" him? You should hurry up and marry him before someone else swipe him. He is a good catch. Why are you wasting time in Jamaica and di man miss you in Boston?"]

Seeing the merit of her concerns, my fiancé and I decided to reduce our expenditures of going back and forth between Boston and Jamaica. We put plans in place for me to join my fiancé in Boston. Naturally, I stopped in Florida to see my daughter and grandchildren. We had a fantastic time together, entertaining, shopping, decorating, and spoiling my grandchildren. However, when it was time to move to Boston, she threw a fit that everyone could remember in our circle. It was hostile, loud, and disrespectful. Even though she encouraged the move, she could not bear that her mother was moving so far away. Because of the fight, we stopped speaking for a while. She later cried, apologized for her behavior, and begged my forgiveness. Thank God we both forgave each other. Two weeks later, Georgia was dead, and none of the fights we had mattered then. Even as I cried, she was so dramatic that I knew I would miss her opinionated honesty, which she shared in heightened anger.

> *"Who will I fight with now? I would rather have a thousand fights with my daughter and have her alive than lying in this casket."*

I wept by that casket until my tear bag was dry. I was drenched in tears as I sat there as if a piece of me had departed, and I too had no life left. The reality of the rest of my life had started to sink in. We had planned to grow old together—where was my daughter? The "How?" "Why?" "Who?" "What?" "When?" "Where?" questions flooded into my spirit. The questions never honestly go away—they only get quieter with passing days and years.

True to form, Georgia made friends just as quickly as I did. She had a terrific group of friends from elementary and high schools who were like daughters to me. Georgia assigned roles to various friends. Nyocca had the role of godmother, a position she continues to serve judiciously in that capacity today. After the burial, Georgia's friends decided to have a repast like none other. They rented a ballroom at a local hotel which they decorated in red, black, and white. They framed trendy pictures and created an elegant, fashionable atmosphere—indeed a celebration of life. They played her favorite music and shared stories about her life and adventures. In keeping with her love of performing arts, her friends performed a beautiful creative dance recital. They role-played some of her hilariously dramatic encounters at school, home, and work. They shared her mischievously cunning satirical escapades.

Combining tears and laughter, we consoled ourselves for a few hours. This event is how Georgia would have planned the celebration of her life. While it was a sad occasion, I believe that the celebration of her short, eventful life was more healing than focusing on how she died. Observing, listening, crying, and laughing through the stories retold by her friends was sincerely inspirational. I took comfort in the way she positively impacted the lives of others.

For a while, my home in Boston was not without a friend or two staying one week, a whole month, or several months at a time.

> *"Those who could not visit sent their love, packages, and prayers. I could feel inner peace when the village knelt to pray on our behalf."*

One of my friends stayed with me until Mother's Day. That was an unwelcome *first, as I knew it would be painful.* Although I had two children that I loved equally, Georgia was my emotional child who celebrated and made a big deal about everything in life. Our first birthday without Georgia, and every birthday since, my family, including her children, unite to light a red candle in her honor. We put her pictures, birthday cake, and fruit juice on the table to celebrate her life. As much as Georgia loved to entertain, she did not drink alcohol.

Despite the five-year age difference, my grandchildren Najja and Nia love and protect each other. My granddaughter Nia was young when her mother died. However, like Georgia's maternal claim on me the day she emerged into the world, Nia's relationship with her mother is intact. No one can usurp Georgia's short role as her birth mother. That is a bond formed nearly ten months before birth and one and a half years after birth.

As the children's mother, Georgia did not want her children raised separately. Their father honored that promise as best as he could. As experience shows, our shared love for Georgia and the children supersedes differences of opinion.

> *"Collectively, both families have gotten better at dealing with disagreements. When we hit deadlocks, as is customary when people grieve, we fight and shout at the unfairness of it all."*

We quickly change our stance to embrace our common purpose. We try not to take our remaining loved ones for granted. Disagreements are handled effectively and not out of proportion. Together, we continue to contribute to the healthy growth and development of Georgia's children.

I am proudly declaring that I brought a lovely human being into this world. She was a bright light that shone in the lives that she touched. She loved her family unconditionally because she knew love. She had a temper that would flare up to a boiling point in a minute, yet she held no festering malice.

> *"The same person who gave you her strong opinions one minute would not hesitate to help you in the next. Georgia gave everything she had, and in the end, she gave her life."*

In her innocence, she could not see the enemy lurking in the wings. When the devil reared its ugly head in her life, and a man shot her to death while her children slept in a room nearby, our entire world spun out of balance.

Since her passing twelve years ago, I have gained strength by pouring my love and energy into her two children—my grandchildren. We keep Georgia's spirit alive with the stories we can share with Najja and Nia. Our shared purpose is to execute their mother's wishes. We find consolation in family rituals, social events, and positive examples shared with the children. Every opportunity I get to go to Florida, I incorporate a visit to her graveside.

> *"Georgia's friends who still live in Florida, including their godmother, Nyocca, also visit her graveside regularly to clean her tombstone, leave red roses, and have conversations with her."*

I have come to appreciate my inner circle friends over the years. I thank God for them every day. I also thank God for the strangers who stop and listen to the stories of my children and grandchildren during my darkest moments.

> *"I am also extremely grateful to their father Trevor, his family, and friends who have been very kind to my grandchildren, helping them to keep their mother's memory alive."*

I pray that my grandchildren will honor their mother's legacy by staying on the right path and doing the right thing. I pray that even during times of sadness, they will pay tribute to her by fulfilling the grand plans she had for them.

As I reflect on my daughter's life, I cannot help but wonder what her life would be like if allowed to live. Life is like a relay race with batons passed among family members. Ultimately, the child must accept the rod, run the leg, finish the race, and claim the victory. Georgia would be proud to know that this book, published twelve years after her death, coincides with Najja's completion of high school and college entrance in Boston (January 2020). Senior year was a season of walking through the blazing fire and refusing to dip in the well. I was reminded of his mother every step of the way. Thank God we had the good sense to join forces to make it happen. It was not an easy road. With the help of the community:

> *"Najja overcame every real or perceived hurdle to complete high school. In the end, he got out of his way and worked diligently and expeditiously to succeed."*

We are confident he will do well regardless of his academic choices. Like Georgia and Trevor, anytime Najja applies himself, he succeeds. Every lesson he learned throughout his eighteen years prepared him for this leg of the race. Georgia would also be happy to know that Nia is living up to her name at thirteen as she explores her purpose. She is intelligent, diligent, bold, conscientious, and has a witty sense of humor. Sounds familiar?

I sometimes reminisce about what Georgia would do or say in a particular situation, and I cannot help but laugh loudly with my head thrown back while thinking, *"This girl is not real."* If there is ever a time that I feel Georgia's presence, it is during challenging times, and when I do, I am comforted. I was despondent that she was not there to witness my wedding to Richard *later that year.* She would be happy to know, *"nobody swiped him from me."* I am even more comforted that she met, evaluated, and loved him despite our initial disagreement.

"She was right—we are perfect for each other. My husband plays the role of an affectionate grandfather to Najja and Nia. They love spending time with him." He is funny because he speaks their language about the latest fashion, bargain hunting, technology, and college.

I get asked all the time if I have any guilt for what happened to my daughter. I respond with a resounding, "NO." Our children will make life choices. In their minds, these choices are best for them. Parents can only pray that ultimately they know what they are doing. I had a close relationship with my child. I miss her terribly. We shared a lot of good memories to keep me going through moments of darkness.

To parents who have never lost a child, no one knows what can happen from one day to the next.

> *"Mend fences quickly because tomorrow is unpromised. When there are disagreements, don't let them fester because of pride and bitterness."*

Remember, in this journey called life, death also comes with it. I am not mourning that she died. I am outraged that someone else tried to play God and deprived us of our ray of sunshine. If we continue to grieve, then the evil one wins. I refuse to say his name as he has no power over us. Let us focus on the positive.

To other parents going through a similar situation, I would say, celebrate your children's life—honor their memory in every possible way you can.

> *"Don't forget the children, spouses, and family members who are still alive." It is easy to lose sight of our loved ones when we grieve."*

Do not dwell on the negative. Pick yourself up and live a little bit extra for the life that went to sleep way too soon.

Reflection Exercise
Deadly Intentions: Georgia Green–Lee's Story

1. *What are your key takeaways from Georgia's story as you struggle with your loss?*	
2. *What instructions do you have for parents experiencing a similar loss?*	
3. *How do you overcome challenges when grief becomes messy within the family unit?*	
4. *How can you help yourself and others work through grief?*	
5. *What advice do you have for strengthening the family unit during grief?*	
6. *List examples of ways you can honor your loved ones(s)*	

CHAPTER 10: GRIEF NEVER ENDS

Grief is synonymous with bereavement—defined as deep feelings of sadness, anguish, heartache, pain, and misery after losing someone to death. After a significant loss, it is evident that grief has no standard, model, or framework upon reviewing each person's experience. Each person addresses sorrow in different ways. Whether a parent is mourning the loss of a baby, teenager, or adult child, the consensus is that parents should not have to bury their children. They should not have to experience such grief. A person's grief is further compounded by how family and friends manage, interpret, or relate to the immediate family's needs.

One contributor suggested that people behaved strangely and awkwardly in her presence as if they did not know what to say. Family and friends try not to say the wrong things. They sometimes try too hard to avoid speaking the child's name as they are overtly mindful of emotional triggers. Yet, as one parent indicated, saying the child's name is their way of honoring the beauty he brought into their lives.

After going through five phases of grief: denial, anger, bargaining, depression, and acceptance, pain, anguish, longing, regret, anxiety, and regurgitation of the last event will continue. A Yale study conducted in 2007 validated five overarching stages of grief: disbelief, yearning, anger, depression, and acceptance.

> *"Yearning or missing a loved one is a more dominant emotion than depression—meaning mental health experts who treat the grief-stricken may need to refocus on feelings of loss." (Kotulak, 2007)*

Grief manifests in physical, mental, behavioral, socio-cultural, sacred, spiritual, and philosophical ways. Within these dimensions are sub-cultural levels and rituals. Except for Melanie's mother, Mimi Cargill, born in Brazil, all the contributors are from Jamaica. However, culture does not prevent them from sharing different ancestral and other sub-cultural ways that grief shows up.

In some cases, people question faith in a higher purpose and, after many tumultuous experiences, have to rebuild that faith. They have to give themselves time to move from disbelief and denial to acceptance. Mark you, acceptance does not mean they will fully overcome grief. It only means they develop additional coping mechanisms.

Scholarly research with a population sample of 1,581 respondents, of which 641 were African Americans, indicates that African Americans grieve differently than their Caucasian counterparts. Overall, African Americans demonstrated greater *complexity* in the grieving process.

> *"African-Americans experience more frequent bereavement by homicide, maintenance of a stronger continuing bond with the deceased, greater grief for the loss of extended kin beyond the immediate family, and a sense of support in their grief, despite their tendency to talk less with others about the loss or seek professional support for it." (Laurie and Neimeyer, 2008)*

Family and friends need to lean into this concept without projecting a set standard or framework for grieving. Since cultural groups are far from consistent, personal deviations are standard. Sub-culture plays a significant role during bereavement. In the case of my brother, Cleveland ("Fox') Nooks, my brother Paul called me at work with the bad news. While my colleagues may have found it shortsighted to give me bad news at work, my close family ties would never forgive someone who withheld such information until after work. Each sibling has cohort support for the bad news. You get bad news; you call your support sibling immediately.

We live in a culture where we do not always know how to approach grief. The messages we send indicate that the sooner one gets back to the ordinary course of their lives, the better one will feel. Our culture of *"the show must go on"* does not always support grieving. People who are suffering will tell you precisely what you want to hear. They do not want you to worry or demonstrate insincere concern. The adoration shown by the children we lose helps to console us. Yet, other triggers send parents in a debilitating emotional frenzy. Annette Nalty wrote about triggers:

> *Smelling Corey's favorite cologne passing the places they visited together, going to the computer repair shop*

We can find solace by hearing how others manage a child's loss—during this stage, listening and observing help both parties. All parents have high hopes and expectations for their children. Some may be comfortable as long as children call home regularly and visit a few times a year. Other parents expect children to complete high school, go to college, get a career, get married, and have children. When a parent loses a child, all those expectations evaporate in thin air. The parents grieve that the child may not have found their true authentic self— there was not enough time. You will recall Dennis Anonymous was in a hurry to experience everything life had to offer. He started various activities well before traditional norms. He drove a car when he was nine years old and had his first car accident at fourteen or fifteen. His mother takes comfort because the urgency he demonstrated as a child allowed him to experience many things. However, not much consolation, this new understanding is only a small step to healing and mending. Recognizing that tomorrow is not guaranteed, parents who experience loss find ways to live in the moment. They remind those who have never experienced anything as devastating to be more thoughtful, loving, forgiving, and supportive.

When songwriter and singer Eric Clapman's four-year-old son, Connor, fell from a 53rd story window in New York City, it was a devasting tragedy. If you recall where you stood when this event occurred, you can still feel chills and pain for the child and his family. How does a parent survive such a dramatic tragedy? Clapton reports that he had experienced grief before when he lost his grandfather. He had contemplated borrowing harmonies from Jamaican-born Jimmy Cliff's song, "*Many Rivers to Cross*," as a way to grieve.

When Clapton lost his precious child, he said he wrote the song "*Tears in Heaven*" as a meditative lyric to keep himself from going crazy during what he described as the darkest period of his life. He used his musical talent and advocacy to heal. As Hyacinth Blake wrote in her tribute to Renee, you do not overcome the loss of your child as long as you are alive. You find better ways to manage the emotional pain. Researchers suggest that parents who are stuck in disbelief, anger, or bargaining beyond six months should seek professional help. Healing and transformation require comprehensive techniques that often challenge us to rise stronger.

> *Changing is not just changing the things outside of us. First of all, we need the right view that transcends all notions, including being and non-being, creator and creature, mind and spirit. That kind of insight is crucial for transformation and healing." (Thich Nhat Hanh). www.awakeningthegreatnesswithin.com)*

CHAPTER 11: GRIEF'S TOLL ON THE FAMILY UNIT

People grieve differently, and grief within family units often takes different turns. It is imperative for parents grieving for children to remember to reconnect with family members left behind—especially spouses and children. Since people suffer in diverse ways, we make assumptions about how people should act in professional settings. These assumptions can lead to incorrect beliefs and devastating outcomes. Some families never emotionally recover from the aftermath of losing a child. Parents may appear emotionally absent as they deal with the loss of children.

There are times when survivor siblings grieve on their own. They sometimes feel emotionally abandoned by parents who are dealing with their pain. They find it challenging to communicate with parents working through their prescribed phases of grief. Families have a difficult time reforming the team dynamics without their *loved* ones. To some extent, perceived blame from all parties involved may deem some relationships irretrievably broken.

It is common for women to accept that their spouses do not support them after losing a child. The men believe that how they deal with grief is often misunderstood by their spouses and friends. In an online publication titled, *Gender Differences in Grief*, Thomas Bekkers, MSW, APSW purports that men grieve much differently than women (October 2013). They do not want to appear weak, so they tend to suppress their feelings and *emotions*. The story of the loss plays over and over in their heads. Vocalizing it to others conjures up more discomfort and pain. Research also confirms that both men women may find external outlets to deal with the pain.

Men often explore new roles or immerse themselves in various non-traditional activities if they lose a spouse and become a single parent. In some cases, women do not understand how men grieve and incorrectly interpret their actions. They see men's reactions as emotionless, detached, or distant. While women co-author this book about losing a child or loved one, the stories are instructional to both men and women. The family unit, generally perceived as team-oriented, is where each person plays a key role. When a member leaves the team, the remaining members must reform—restructuring roles and responsibilities. The loss is sometimes difficult on the remaining members as they must learn how to manage without their loved ones.

There is also the extreme case of a spouse waking from a coma to realize that of the five people traveling in a car that day, he or she is the only member alive. Every member of his or her immediate family is deceased in a matter of minutes, and with them, all their dreams and aspirations. There must be prolonged feelings of disconnection, despair, sorrow, loneliness, isolation, and frustration. It is not uncommon for the survivor to turn his or her ire on other extended family members.

> *"Our dead are never dead to us until we have forgotten them"*
> *(George Eliot)*

Any disagreements or challenges that existed before the accident now multiplied exponentially. Blame gets tossed back and forth, especially when hopelessness replaces faith. It often takes years, if ever, for such relationships to Meanwhile, survivors often left alone to fill all the roles previously fulfilled by former members feel overwhelmed. During these times, recipients of such wrath must exercise mindfulness--silencing the mind, listening to the heart, and finding hurt where it dwells. For some people, it means meditation and for others finding your center in physical activities such as yoga, stretching, dancing, or swimming. Mindfulness is about self-awareness, social awareness, empathy, love, patience, and understanding.

> *"In order to overcome challenges in messy situations with family members, it is okay to step away from them. Space and time will*

> *allow for healing, understanding, and acceptance." (Sharon Carter, 2020)*

According to the Mayo Clinic on grieving, writing these stories can evoke grief even years after the event occurred. When I wrote my brother's stories and edited the others, I felt empathy for my parents and friends who sacrificed so much and lost so much. Writing the tribute to their children must have reopened their wounds well beyond my imagination. Even though the annual rituals bring some comfort, include joyful memories to keep spirits optimistic and hopeful.

> *"For the Spirit God gave us does not make us timid, but gives us power, love, and self-discipline" (2 Timothy 1:7: NIV)*

CHAPTER 12: HOW TO SUPPORT GRIEF STRICKEN PARENTS

This book is a celebration of life rather than a commemoration of death. It is a remarkable truth that I hold dear as a commentator of the human condition: ***"In the middle of life, life happens."*** The end is never timely, and with death, age is just a number. I remember a friend of mine cuddling the very slender frame of her grandmother, who was ninety-three-years-old. I enjoyed the weekends I accompanied them to buy eggs and milk from the farm in Maine's countryside. My friend whimpered like a baby after her grandmother had the stroke. Her grandmother was a lovely lady with a strong mental capacity and a terrific host. No matter where I was in the world when she answered the phone, our conversations always left me smiling.

Standing by the hospital bed that morning, I was at a loss for words. I kept thinking, *"She lived a long life. Perhaps, she is tired and ready to go."* Much to my delight, her granddaughter, her caregiver, nursed her back to health. She enjoyed another thirteen or so years on this earth. Just imagine the trauma experienced by a parent who loses a child who did not get a chance to experience life to the fullest. It is indeed unbearable for family and friends experiencing such a horrific loss. Many people in the work environment are at a loss for words when dealing with a grief-stricken colleague. Their first instinct is to console the colleague. However, after slowly evaluating many communication filters: culture, customs; language; values; personality; ties; and age of the deceased, coworkers would rather skip into an empty office to avoid making a blunder. Below are a few statements by parents and contributors who returned to work after losing a child:

> *"I wish they never said, "he is in a better place" or ask how it happened. I would have preferred if they had just given me a hug and said nothing because there is nothing they could have said to make me feel better" (Ingrid Anonymous).*

> *"They were very understanding. I told them if they see me crying, I am okay because there are days when that is going to happen" (Valerie Shelton).*

> *"I was self-employed, working for Rachel Williams. She gave me a whole month off. It was crying time. I needed it. I returned to work part-time at the beginning of January 2013" (Mimi Cargill)*

> *"As you can imagine, the phone kept ringing off the hook. Grief struck me like a ton of bricks. I was inconsolable and could not speak to anyone though I could surely feel their prayers" (Sharon Carter).*

While a parent is grieving for his or her child, colleagues may have a strong desire for things to return to "normal." Rest assured, things may never return to normal for that person, as grief never ends. Colleagues mean well when they try to find a quick solution for a grieving parent. They often make assumptions that the quicker one gets back to work, the better. Do not make assumptions that you know how someone feels during this challenging period. Even if you lost a child, each situation is unique. People find solace in different ways. Below is a heartbreaking question on Facebook from a father who lost his teenage son recently:

> *"How do I find peace?" (Anonymous)*

I do not know the gentleman personally. I was in the middle of capturing the stories for this book when his tragedy occurred. I ache for the parents who lost a teenaged son with a promising future. Although we can channel our responses based on his profile, nothing will suffice at this early grieving stage. He is yet another bereaved parent who lost a son to gun violence. Gun violence of any kind from anyone is just that—brutality. In the meantime, how do we protect our loved ones from these and other brutal assaults? Who is next?

Grief often stands at our door and demands answers to these questions. How will we respond? There are no "right words" to say to a grieving parent. Even if the person is a close friend, it is not easy to figure out what to say. Observing and listening are terrific strategies. Do not ignore the fact that your colleague has experienced a significant loss. In his or her mind, the emotional assault may be permanent. Do not be afraid to acknowledge the loss and offer condolences.

> *".............Still, others just acted as nothing had happened. Those people irritated me the most as it seems that they were discounting this precious life. But again, I realize that it is difficult to know how to console someone on such a significant loss (Annette M. Nalty).*

There is that nagging temptation to make a long speech to cover uncomfortable silence. Restraint feels awkward, especially when everyone is reeling from the loss. Find out from the person how you can help—what support is needed.

> *Having walked the plank, I now have a better understanding that, in general, people mean well. There are no words sufficient to console a grieving parent. However, merely acknowledging the loss with "I am sorry" goes a long way" (Annette Nalty).*

It is just heartbreaking that so many of my friends experienced substantial losses. Understanding the dynamics of the relationship with the *bereaved* parents is extremely important. It is also essential to understand the culture of the grieving family. Except for Mimi Cargill and Sharon Carter, all the book contributors are friends I met at work more than forty years ago. In Mimi Cargill's Brazilian culture, the funeral takes place almost immediately after death. When a person dies in Jamaica, as was the case with my brother Cleveland, funeral services could be several weeks after death. There are many evening events (nine nights) where the community celebrated his life up to the night before the burial. Everyone needs time to make travel arrangements from several countries. The period between passing and funeral is shorter when it occurs in the United States. When tragedy strikes a community, there is an outpouring of support from family and strangers. Everyone is thinking: *"It could have been my family or me."* It is a community of people working towards a common goal.

We make every effort to support our friends in whatever capacity they will allow. For example, when Annette Nalty called to tell me about the accident that took Beth Wilson–Smalling's brother and three nephews in Pennsylvania almost seventeen years ago, I was lost and could not function. It was a terrible blow to the family and community of friends. I was in Indianapolis, Indiana, USA, on an assignment and was due to fly back to Maine,

USA, where I lived. I could not change the flight to go to Atlanta as airfares were costly back then. Emergency travel was expensive. I took a Greyhound Bus and traveled all night to get to Atlanta, Georgia. I have some peculiar stories about that transportation experience, which has to stay for another time. Meanwhile, Annette and her husband traveled from South Carolina to Atlanta, Georgia. Beth and her younger brother, Dean, drove all night from New York City to Atlanta to meet me at the Greyhound Bus station downtown.

Although the funeral had already taken place in New York, we just had to be there to support our friends. That weekend we did not speak much about the tragedy. We were still in shock. We cooked, wept, laughed, and whimpered while Dane, former spouse and consummate host, played reggae music to boost our spirits. When Beth had a painful moment, we gave her time and space. When she returned to work, she was pleasantly surprised by the support she received from her coworkers and supervisors.

I was heading to Hilton Head, South Carolina, to facilitate a 5-day MBA workshop when I heard about Corey's passing. I pulled over by the side of the road, as I was too shocked to drive. My body shook with tears for a long time. He was our *first baby*—the first among the group of friends. This time it was Beth who shared the distressing news. Several of our close friends assembled at home that weekend to support them. Friends and coworkers of the grieving couple often visited to drop off food, cards, and flowers.

When Hyacinth lost her daughter, Renee, we all traveled from different parts of the country to support the family a few years later. We are former coworkers who remained connected over the years. Our social ties, which started in the workplace, stay strong. Our family-oriented values and love for each other remain strong.

When Mrs. SD, a former work colleague we met more than forty years ago, lost her daughter in 2019, about eleven of us attended the funeral. Those who could not make it sent prayers; warm, affectionate thoughts; cards; flowers; texts, declarations, commendations, or post sincere condolences on social media.

When there is a fallen soldier or officer, people come from far and wide to honor the fallen soldier or officer. The work environment should not be any different. The bereaved may ask for time off from work to support the distant family or grieving friends. While it may not be a blood relative, strong cultural and community-based ties bind us together across land and sea. Being present to support the family and close friends is essential.

I was heading to Orlando for a seminar when Beth and Annette called about the sudden passing of Hyacinth Blake's daughter, Renee. After we digested the distressing news quietly, we each sprang into action. We all agreed to meet at my hotel and drive to Hyacinth's home that Friday. Beth drove in from Atlanta, GA, and we attended the funeral. During the days following the news and the funeral, it was evident that the arrival of several other friends and coworkers made a huge difference.

Managers and supervisors have to understand that grief does not end when the funeral finishes. It is just the beginning. Empathizing with the bereaved demonstrates social awareness and leads to better relationships. Any parent whose child has had a "near-death" experience understands the terrible feeling of relief that the child survived the event. Think about how anxious you were when that happened. Now, think about the child who did not make it. Think about how that parent feels.

> *"I thought I was going crazy."* Eric Clapton

There is nothing we can say that will bring the child back. However, one mother felt comfortable, knowing that her inner circle friends were praying for her. Once you know and understand your grieving colleague's needs, you are more likely to respond appropriately. Grieving parents find creative ways to deal with emotional ups and downs that come crashing out of nowhere, hitting them like a migraine on steroids.

> *During my darkest days, I relied heavily on my fiancé, family, and friends. An encouraging telephone call could make a difference in how I felt that day. Words of comfort and support made such a huge difference during my time of enormous grief"* (Sharon Carter, 2020).

Research shows that grief is often messy. Bereaved parents experience emotional lows leading to raw, self-preserving vulnerability. Their biggest fear is sharing the bitterness of openness to the world. How will it be used against them now or in the future?

Solitude exacerbates shame, anxiety, fear, agony, and hopelessness. Your grieving colleague may also be experiencing difficulties reconciling the aftermath at home. They may be involved in self-blame, being blamed, or blaming others. If you feel cornered at home in your grief, seek resources at work or through other external channels. Suppose you are a supervisor and observe an employee struggling for an extended period after a significant loss. In that case, it is okay to refer the employee to available resources he or she may have overlooked (e.g., employee assistance programs). Please keep in mind that not every culture feels comfortable with external counseling. On the same trend, interactions with objective outsiders are the right strategies for the bereaved. Both counselor and employee should have an initial meeting where mutual evaluation and "good fit" conversations occur.

Immediately after the employee returns to work, managers need to exercise social awareness. Do not assume that a lighter workload is appropriate as the person may view work as a valuable distraction. Asking questions is a sure way to gain a better understanding of your employee's current needs. Read both body language and voice intonations. It is easy to miss the real meaning of: *"I am okay!" "No problem, mans!" I will get it done!"* Do not forget to look for signs that indicate, "I need help!"

> *"Bereaved parents think of "1,001 firsts" after the passing of a child. If they decide to take a day off on the anniversary of his or her birthday and the day of the child's passing, please understand that decompressing is an integral part of grieving" (Dr. Pauline E. Wallner, Nee Nooks).*

Reflection Exercise
A Love Letter

'Mimi' Cargill wrote a love letter to her daughter, which she rereads to comfort her in times of stress and loneliness. When you are ready, write a love letter to your child. Start with a couple of paragraphs:

Each time you have an emotional meltdown or a joyful reason, add to the love letter. Feel free to use the blank pages provided at the end of the book to write the letter or start a journal. If you are in a support group or subscribe to a magazine, share your letter with other parents experiencing a similar loss.

Reflection Exercise
A Love Letter

When you are ready, try writing a love letter to your child. Start with a couple of paragraphs:

Each time you have an emotional low or a joyful reason, add to the love letter. Feel free to use the blank pages provided at the end of the book to write the letter or start a journal. If you are in a support group or subscribe to a magazine, share your letter with other parents experiencing a similar loss

> *"Quit thinking that you know how someone feels or how they should prioritize their lives after a significant loss. Reflect on three key take-a-ways: life is short; engage each other with love; leave no reasons for regret."*
> (Dr. Pauline E. Wallner, D.M)

CHAPTER 13: THE OVERARCHING LESSONS ON GRIEVING

Cleveland G. Nooks, Corey O. Nalty, and Dennis Anonymous gravitated towards people who struggled with finding their rightful place in society. They demonstrated compassion for the underdog and wanted the absolute best for them. They showed a certain level of understanding that perplexed parents, causing them to scratch their heads in wonder. Interestingly, this sentiment, expressed by people who experienced grief and wrote about it, provides insights into grief.

At the end of a Fall 2019 seminar designed for corporate controllers in Washington, DC, I learned about a book titled *Color Him Father* (Drake II, 2017)—written by grieving fathers. Drake II touchingly outlined his daughter's life as a way of expressing his grief, helping other fathers to do the same. His daughter considered him an exemplary father. As such, whenever she encountered friends or associates she believed would benefit from her father's wise counsel, she either brought them home or encouraged him to speak to them (Drake II, 2017). His book addresses the way fathers deal with grief. I recommend this body of work for parents who encountered suffering or are seeking to support others. The women who shared their stories in this book also provided critical lessons for grieving parents that I summarized below:

The Power of Prayer

During various phases of grief, we often have conversations with someone or something outside of ourselves. In a state of disbelief, we shout and curse the "evil one." We also turn our "Why" questions to a higher power we describe as *God the Father*, Lord, Master, *Jesus the Son*, *Holy Spirit*, *Jehovah*: *(Prophet*; *Jireh*; *Nissi*, *Makadesh)*, *Allah*, *Elohim*, *Yahweh*, *El Shaddai*, *Adonai*. It is never initially clear to us why things happen the way they do. Deep down, we hope our feelings of loss and initial indescribable grief will go away.

All the contributors in this book found comfort in their faith, regardless of religious affiliations. Within faith-based homes, it is crucial to recognize that families and friends have different perceptions about religion, prayer, and dedication during grief. For example, Hyacinth Blake, like many others, cherishes her relationship with God. This form of faith is more authentic and acceptable to her than organized religion. Although she does not subscribe to an established religion, she walks and talks with God all day long.

Sometimes, we are so angry and lonely that praying becomes difficult. Occasionally, we distance ourselves from conversations with God *because* our grief is so intense. Even people who do not share the same religious beliefs find comfort in praying for each other. When family, friends, and *"prayer groups"* petition the Lord on our behalf, we often feel comforted. Whatever struggles we go through, there is solace in prayer. In intercessory prayer, there is power said, contributor Sharon Carter,

> *"I was comforted when I knew that people were praying for us."*

Prayer stabilizes fear and anxiety. In a recent video post on Facebook, Steve Harvey, comedian, author, producer, television, radio, and game show host, strongly emphasized, *"Prayer changes things."*

No matter who we are, grief is a common factor in our lives—all of us have experienced grief somehow. We must remember, however, that each person must seek a relationship with God. Such a relationship grows stronger through prayer and study. Although God knows our heart's desires, he wants to hear directly from us as we worship him during good and bad times. Praying is so challenging when grief bleeds into the spirit and pushes joy out. As Annette Nalty stated when she wrote about losing Corey:

> *"I found it difficult to pray. I was mad at God. How could he take him now that he was getting his life together and reaping the benefits of all his earlier struggles." (Annette P. Nalty)*

Annette voiced this opinion to her church pastor. He told her not to stop talking to God.

> *"If you can't voice your sorrow to God, who else can you take it to?"*

Despite the questioning tone when having conversations with God, the line of communication is still open. Having faith for things unseen requires courage. That personal interaction with God produces a discerning spirit that leads to peace. Many people believe that prayer must be in a religious prose book, including formal language and being sanctimoniously grand. Others believe that an informal, ordinary conversation with God is okay. Although there is no set standard for grief, the women expressed times when faith, hope, and love replaced the terrible, aching assault of grief. Mimi Cargill writes about her unwavering faith in God when her grief in losing Melanie set in like a robber of peace.

> *"God has a way of keeping things simple for us. From the day we are born, we start to die. I am glad that Melanie embraced the beauty of God's Holy Spirit even during her darkest challenges."*
> *(Mimi Cargill)*

The author of *"The Power of a Praying Wife*, Stormie Omartian, reminds us that as we go through emotional turmoil, prayer is the perfect petition for healing and cleansing the soul from negative thoughts and actions. We do not always know why things happen. However, we know that when bad things happen, we can seek comfort in God's promises.

> *"Do not be anxious about anything, but in everything by prayer and supplication with thanksgiving, let your requests be made known to God. And the peace of God which surpasses all understanding will guard your hearts and your minds in Christ Jesus." (Philippians 4: 6-7 - NIV)*

Perspectives & Pride

Research indicates that men and women approach grief differently. One family member or spouse may seek answers and support through various external channels. Other family members or spouses may believe that dwelling on grief may be a sign of weakness. Women sometimes describe their spouses as withdrawn, unavailable, emotionless, or sedentary after losing a child. Different perspectives and complexities lead to many inferences, followed by miscommunication, erroneous beliefs, and irretrievable separations among family members. These events occur with both spouses and children.

Grief does not discriminate—it affects us all. We use our experience to help us ride the "roller coasters" that phases of grief throw at us. In October 2019, Christian recording artist TobyMac and his wife Amanda lost their first-born son. He was an aspiring rapper who was only twenty-one years old. TobyMac stated that losing his son is by far the most painful experience to date. He released a new song in his son's honor, *"Twenty-one years,"* asking the same question that so many of the contributors asked:

> *"..........................Why would you give him and take him away?"*

This love song demonstrates the immeasurable faith of someone grieving the loss of a child. He sings about his twenty-one years of blessings, though temporary.

> *"......God has you in heaven, but I have you in my heart,".... "Did you wrap him up inside your arms to let him know he is home?" He thanks God for loaning him his son for twenty-one years"* (TobyMac, 2019)

Valerie Shelton expressed a similar sentiment in her story about Wayne. She writes about her 34-year gift.

There are times when *"If"* starts every sentence, a hazardous phase when grieving. Ultimately, someone in the family receives blame for doing something to contribute to the deadly outcome. Some of the domino effect of miscommunication after a loss comes from personal pride, blame, and hopelessness. It is not unusual for people going through grief to replay life-altering events repeatedly, recreating them into more palatable scenarios.

It is also quite common for the finger to point inward. This practice is no less dangerous than blaming someone else. Pride is at the core of wrecked relationships. When disasters happen, pain cloaks grief into rags of pride and a fierce desire to be right. Blame and finger-pointing leave no room for forgiveness and reconciliation. Acting like a dagger, pride sharpens pangs of grief. Sometimes, parental strategies differ after losing a loved one. Families must seek to bridge perceived or real conflicts by resolving issues before it is too late.

> *"Pride goes before destruction, a haughty spirit before a fall"* (Proverbs 16:18-NIV).

A professional mediator during these difficult challenges can defuse tension and strife. Even within congenial environments, families do have financial, emotional, and spiritual disputes. If there are financial disputes, do not wait until they are severe to seek help. Investigate all resources available to you and your family. Remember, forgiveness is healthy for all parties:

> *Forgiveness is a deliberate, authentic, positive, and healthy action that requires a change in mindset towards an offender. Forgiveness occurs when the wronged individual decides to release all ill feelings towards the perpetrator as a means of living a healthier life. (Dr. Pauline E. Wallner, Nee Nooks)*

Passion and Purpose

Vision is the aspiration, desire, target, goal, or objective to which all tangible and intangible resources are retrieved and allotted. A person's mission is a primary reason for existence. Mission-driven individuals and families formulate, exhibit, and live their purpose. Although not many people have a formal mission statement, it is evident in the way they live. The mission is the reason behind dedication to a cause—meaningful actions, initiatives, measures, and outcomes that solidify a lifelong legacy. The purpose is an ambition that keeps the body at a high temperature, the heart pulsating vigorously, and the body in sync. When a decease's vision is executed by remaining loved ones, healing occurs.

The children featured in this book made plans and lived as if they were here before. More importantly, they did not waiver from their dreams. They reminded family members about their passion and purpose. They attacked life with impatience and foresight. They had little patience for anyone who did not see things their way. It leaves us to wonder if somehow they knew, perhaps subconsciously, that their lifespan was short. Annette Nalty recalled her son's dream in which he saw his tombstone, and though he did not identify the date of his passing, he knew he had not reached age thirty. This phenomenon is not easy to explain. This dream, however, was somewhat reassuring. Be mindful that her reality may not be your experience. Search your heart and find what works for you.

Children resist any interference from parents concerning personal and career aspirations. Wayne loved motorcycles. He loved to ride and bought two motorcycles without telling his parents. He also volunteered as a "Big Brother." Georgia visualized two children in her future and built her life strategy around that goal. Corey and Christopher had setbacks and fought profusely and diligently to reinvent themselves. Jason, a dear friend of Dennis, moved from a precarious city to seek stability in another. They were young men just starting to experience and enjoy their lives. They were out celebrating their birthdays. Just as things seemed to be going well, disaster struck. Perhaps, Renee chose a career of caring for others because her respiratory issues increased empathy for others in similar situations.

> *"The fear of death follows from the fear of life. A man who lives fully is prepared to die at any time." Mark Twain (www.brainyquote.com)*

Parents who lose children do things that keep their vision alive through their siblings, grandchildren (if any), or communities. Hyacinth Blake and Annette Nalty continue to explore ways to channel pain by helping others. Ingrid Anonymous spends quality time with her grandchildren and remaining children. Sharon Carter pours Georgia's vision into her children, Najja and Nia, and her remaining daughter, Jeniel. She also spends valuable time with Georgia's childhood friends and their families. Valerie Shelton and her family maintain relationships with Wayne's friends. Some create family and friends' reunions because they now recognize that life is fragile. They no longer postpone opportunities to travel, socialize, and enjoy life.

Okay, so here is where you will ask me about affordability or economic means. I know some people cannot afford any of these suggestions. However, look for activities in your local community that are free or come at a minimal cost. If you do not have a church family, find one. Attending church is not merely about religion—it is about love, fellowship, and survival. People need people. Church folks generally take care of members and neighbors. If you are a single parent who has ever spent a night in a hospital and has no visitors, you will understand this sentiment. The right church family will advocate for you in times of distress.

Veterans join their associations for support and to expand their network. Visit a breakfast or lunch meeting at a Rotary Club, Kiwanis, or Lion's Club any day of the week. Listen keenly to the testimonials given by club members. It is incredible what a small group of people can accomplish when they pool resources.

Search for local walk/run events or even train for a marathon. These physical activities in your child's name bring light into the lives of parents and families. I have a select group of friends that are at my doorstep at the drop of a hat. When they call, I drop what I am doing, and I respond. Who are the people in your circle? Are you shutting them out of your life because you do not want to talk about your feelings? Do you know of anyone who experienced a recent loss? Your experience may help save a life.

Singers write songs to heal themselves and others while preventing mental breakdown. Poets often write sonnets to maintain a positive attitude—taking it one day at a time. In this book, the grieving parents exhibited passion and purpose by keeping their children alive in loving stories. A couple of the contributors frequently speak about writing love letters to their children. If parents had the power to do it all over again, they would change so many things. Although you cannot change your child's past or circumstances, you can slowly start living again. Learn from their experience and honor your children and family as you see fit.

Remember, today's feelings are not permanent—replace them with beautiful memories. In the cruel journey of grief, we are not alone. Do something you have always wanted to do. Join a *painting* workshop, travel to places your children wanted to see, or take up gardening or join an acting class. How about yoga, meditation, bird watching? I saw a group of US/EU residents bird watching—of all places, in the Blue Mountain Hills of Portland, Jamaica. These are the hills where "*real Jamaican coffee*" is grown and exported. If you are lucky to be at the local brewery, you will experience coffee brewed over an open fire and served in a traditional enamel mug. I visited that terrain with my hiking friend about fifteen months ago to formulate my vision and enjoy the mountain air. That day, I listened to the water running behind the trees and enjoyed the nostalgic sounds of birds singing softly. Sounds too idyllic or expensive? How about a greyhound bus to Maine, Florida, or Georgia? You can create similar experiences all year long, depending on your favorite season. The objective is to get out of your comfort zone and try something different. Joining or forming a local outdoor club is also helpful.

There you go again, wanting to throw the book or, better yet, rotten tomatoes at me. I would be lying if I said I did not care what you think or do. I do care what you think and how I might be trivializing the saddest time of your lives. If any of these instructions seem trifling, start by acknowledging the absurdity of my advice. However, understand that a conversation with any of the contributors would reveal similar exploits, applied to bring harmony. Good, let us review some examples:

Annette Nalty and her husband find solace in fishing expeditions, enjoying the stillness of the seas. Remember that when the storm raged on the ocean and the boat was about to capsize, it was Jesus who said, "Peace be still." While it may mean nothing to you, it is quality time engaged in an activity they both enjoy. Even if one spouse dislikes the chosen activity, supporting the other keeps the communication open. Mimi Cargill, the mother of Melanie, is completing a bachelor's degree. We have had several humorous moments over the past few months regarding her college experience. She asked me not to mention her age in this forum. She said, *"No matter how good I do, my age is always the benchmark."* She gets a "kick" out of being introduced on campus. Beth Wilson-Smalling completed a formal bachelor's degree about six months ago. I cannot begin to tell you how many people she tutored through college before she took up the challenge herself. She was a considerable help editing this book. Beth has also embarked on a new and exciting journey. Indeed, another terrific example of stepping out of her comfort zone. Sharon Carter spent a whole year planning and completing a summer cruise with family and friends. Hyacinth Blake makes cruising with family look so easy.

Indeed, you cannot get away from your thoughts. However, do what you must to survive. Your family needs you. If you are alone, sponsor or support a child with similar aspirations as your dearly departed child. Take your time and enjoy your journey. Quiet your mind—listen in silence—open your heart. Allow the sweet essence of your child to shine as you continue to represent and advocate for him or her.

Promises and Protection

People who experience challenges and hold on to their faith will tell you:

> *"Our most personal confidant is God. Whatever conversations we have with him stays with him."*

No matter how difficult our journey, God promised that he would never leave us or forsake us during our darkest hour of need. He understands our struggles with grief, and he has the power to protect us from ourselves. When the Psalmist David found himself exiled from Israel and ridiculed by his enemies, he plunged into depression. In Psalm 42:3, David laments:

> *"My tears have been my food day and night. While people say to me all day long. "Where is your God?"*

Though his state of mind was one of desolation, he placed all his hope in God and found peace in praising him.

> *"Be merciful to me LORD, for I am faint; O LORD, heal me, for my bones are in agony. My soul is in anguish." (Psalm 6:2-3-NIV)*

God described Job as blameless—a man of impeccable integrity God knew could withstand the devil's temptations. When Job went through periods of loss, his wife encouraged him to curse God and die. He refused as he knew that God had promised to protect him. The book of Ruth in the Christian bible shares a brief story of Naomi, Ruth's mother-in-law. She lost her husband and her two sons after moving from Judea to Moab. Yet, despite the circumstances and periods of wavering faith, God kept his promises to her and provided for her.

Like David, Job, and Naomi, we often question God's existence when we experience grief and feelings of abandonment, loneliness, or hopelessness. Another friend of mine lost her daughter recently—murdered by someone she knew. Although I cannot get into the details of the subsequent events, what I can say without a shadow of a doubt, is that her professed faith in God has kept her sane. In these stories, we recall God's promises to protect us from our enemies. When we find that we cannot express our anguish or grief using our own words, the Psalmist does it eloquently for us:

> *"The Lord is my light and my salvation—whom shall I fear? The Lord is the stronghold of my life—of whom shall I be afraid?"*
> (Psalm 27:1-NIV)

It is easy to sink into a deep depression after a significant loss, and the temptations of self-harm run rampant. As Sharon A. White-Answer-Carter shared, *"Depression is real in the grieving process."* Before giving up, think about what your child would want. He or she would certainly not want you to live a life of hopelessness. Do not be defeated as you search for answers or seek solace. Do not be afraid to seek help from friends, family, and support groups. In one of Christian singer TobyMac's lyrics, he encourages listeners to:

> *"Stay in the fight until the final round."*

While you will never overcome the loss of your loved ones, you will undoubtedly find peace in knowing that God keeps his *promises* of protection. It is difficult to know when family, friends, and co-workers struggle from depression because they often share a cheerful facade. The outward appearance rarely matches the turmoil that is running a train wreck inside. Research on depression indicates that some people are *high-functioning* depressives. In a HuffPost (Wellness) article titled, *"11 Truths Only People With High Functioning Depression Will Understand,* Nicole Pajer writes:

> *"Most days, you plaster a smile on your face, excel at work, and even maintain successful relationships. This doesn't mean that you are not struggling from the debilitating symptoms of depression each and every day." (Nicole Pajer, 2019)*

If you or a loved one is facing prolonged internal sadness of any kind, seek help immediately. It is always prudent to err on the side of caution. When you experience emotional triggers, and your Amygdala *(the part of the brain that releases fight or flight responses)* is repeatedly proposing adverse reactions, it is judicious to recognize imminent danger. It is time to reexamine damaging temperaments. Change internal conversations to affirm your intentions for a purposeful life. Neither you nor I can change the past. Instead, evaluate options embedded in the concept of "mindfulness," focusing on seeking emotional, physical, spiritual, and psychological balance.

Write your thoughts down as you experience them. Modern technology allows us to record and store ideas and thoughts easily: computers, smartphones, watches, and social media. Take a walk and keep holding your head high so you can take in the view. This strategy is a simple technique to remind yourself you are still here and you are not alone. Find your notepad on your phone and write what you are feeling—good or bad. Journal your moods while searching the scriptures for places where you are called *blessed* and where you are honored.

> *"Blessed are they who grieve for they shall be consoled"*
> *(Matthew 5:4: NIV).*

Okay, before deciding to throw this book at my self-righteously pious advice again, try it first. If you discover that hope gives you a better outlook than hopelessness, then keep looking for answers within and outside of yourself. Grief causes mental instability, and recovery for some people is elusive. Remember, mental illness is color and gender-blind. There is no shame in admitting that you are losing control. I cannot recall who recently stated:

> *"We take good care of ourselves below the neck yet fail to take care of ourselves above the neck." (Unknown).*

It may have been one of the contributors to this book or a TEDx speaker on YouTube. Was it the hilarious comedian and actress Tiffany Haddish? Can we learn anything about mental illness from Jada Pinkett Smith on Red Table Talk, Robin Roberts on ABC, Iyanla Vanzant on OWN, my mother, the man or woman in the street, or all of the above? The reality is that whether rich or poor, employed or unemployed, cash strapped or not, religious or spiritual, we can learn something from everyone.

Take the lessons you can and apply them within the context of your situation. Do not be afraid to question what you are feeling. Honor your feelings appropriately while putting one foot before the other as you walk by faith. Your survival techniques may be different from mine. Ultimately, survival means living one day at a time—moving beyond mere existence—living as you honor your child's life. If you like music, make sure you have your playlist handy. When you feel like crying, do not be pressured by society's timetable and suppress your emotions. Simultaneously, do not be tempted to self-medicate beyond the pain or engage in addictive behaviors.

Know your triggers because they will derail your efforts. Through mindfulness techniques (e.g., meditation, prayer, exercise) and emotional intelligence (awareness of self, others, environment), you will begin to teach those around you to understand your state of mind. You, too, will start to understand the context in which you work and navigate it accordingly.

> *"Whether you are grieving for a child, parent, sibling, nephew, or any loved one, repressing your emotions is ill-advised. By acknowledging what you are feeling, you are honoring your emotions. Stifled emotions feast on your physical well-being and cause pain."*

If you find that you are crying for days on end and cannot stop, reach out to a friend or designated support group—formal or informal. Many of the contributors write of their community of supporters. Do not lock yourself away from everyone. Sure, you need time with your thoughts. However, people need support—especially when they are hurting.

There is no universal way to grieve. There are too many variables. As the women who tell the stories expressed, they are more likely to seek harmony in support groups and honor their loved ones through various activities. They may also continue family rituals to pay tribute to the spirit of their loved ones. Some women become grief advocates and counselors. Others memorialize their loved ones by celebrating birthdays and holidays at their resting places. Some even choose to have regular conversations with their loved ones during those visits. Sharon, Nyocca, and Najja visited Georgia's resting place on January 20, 2020, twelve years after her passing. They cleaned the plaque and laid flowers. It was an emotionally cleansing experience for eighteen-year-old Najja, who is embarking on a new phase in his life.

We hope that you were able to discover that you are not alone in your grief. We pray that your loved ones' precious memories will act as a rejuvenating source of joy and peace, reducing the pain you are now experiencing.

> *Only through the significant loss of my loved ones have I truly begun to live. When their eyes closed, mine opened. (Angie Corbett-Kuiper at www.goodreads.com)*

Keep Rising Stronger™

WALK GOOD!
SAFE TRAVELS!

PERSONAL JOURNAL

PERSONAL JOURNAL:

PERSONAL JOURNAL:

RISING STRONGER SERIES™

PERSONAL JOURNAL:

PERSONAL JOURNAL:

PERSONAL JOURNAL:

PERSONAL JOURNAL:

RISING STRONGER SERIES™

PERSONAL JOURNAL:

PERSONAL JOURNAL:

BIBLIOGRAPHY

Bekkers, T. (2013). Gender differences in grief. BLOG. Green Bay Oncology. www. Gboncology.com

Clements, P. T., et al. (2003). Journal of Psychosocial Nurse Mental Health Service. Nov; 41(11):8 author reply 8-9

Drake II., L. M. (2019). *Color him, father. Brown Girl Books, LLC.* Houston, Texas. Washington, D.C.

Kotulak, R. (2007, Feb 22). *Yale study confirms   validity of long-held 5 stages of grieving; longing for a loved one is found to be a bigger factor than depression—a finding that could help in treatment.:* HOME EDITION]. *Los Angeles Times* Retrieved from https://search.proquest.com/docview/422127 070?accountid=35812

Kubler-Ross, E. & Kessler, D. (2005). *On grief and grieving. Finding the meaning of grief through the five stages of loss.* New York. Toronto. Scribner.

Laurie, A & Neimeyer, R. A. (2008). African Americans in bereavement: Grief as a function of Ethnicity.

Omartian, S. (2012). The power of a praying wife. Hawkins Children's, LLC. Harvest House Publisher's, Inc.

Pajer, N. (2019). *11 truths only people with high functioning depression will understand*, HuffPost (Wellness). (www.huffpost.com).

Pickhardt, Ph.D., C. E. (2009). Rebel with a cause: Rebellion in Adolescence.....and why the antidote is not punishment but real independence. (www.psychologytoday.com)

Sandberg, S., & Grant, A. M. (2017). Option B: Facing adversity, building resilience, and finding Joy). Borzoi Book. Alfred A. Knoph, New York

TobyMac (2019). *Twenty-one years.* www.youtube.com.

Ram Dass. (2012). *A letter to Rachel.* www.ramdass.org.

Wallner, P. E. (2019). Rising Stronger™: Living, Loving, and Leading From a Seat of Gratitude. NMWB Global Management Services, LLC.

(https://www.fromgrieftogratitude.com/

https://www.mayoclinic.org/healthy-lifestyle/end-of-life/in-depth/grief/art-20045340

ABOUT THE BOOK

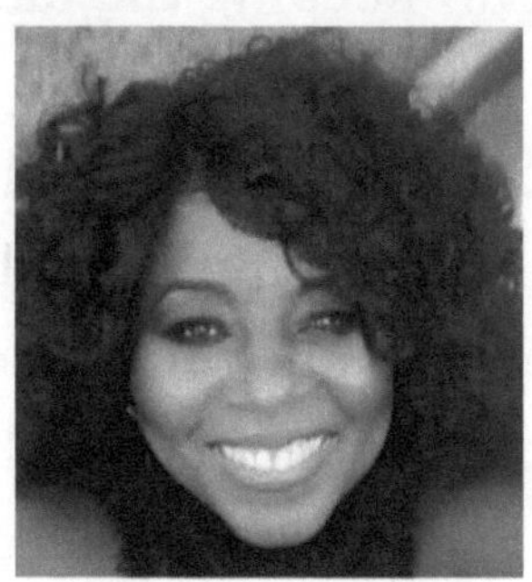

By the time this book is published, it will be the second in the Rising Stronger Series™. The first book in the series: ***Rising Stronger: Living, Loving, and Leading from a Seat of Gratitude***, was published in February 2019. Ever since, and because of the overwhelming response to my first attempt at self-publishing, I have had a strong desire to create a series to help different population segments develop blueprints for Rising Stronger™.

The second book in the Rising Stronger Series™: *Loving and Essential Paths to Healing After Losing a Child*™ is possible through the collaborative efforts of contributors, writers, and editors. The contributors are amazing women I have known or have been in my inner circle for 20–43 years. The stories act as conscious awakenings of love and a heartbreaking reminder of the beautiful lives taken too soon. The co-authors, interconnected by invisible badges of bravery, resilience, and tenacity, share their grief experiences. They live by unquestionable energy and passion for keeping the faces of their children alive.

In doing so, the contributors share how they have been managing their lives after enormous losses. The courage demonstrated by them in allowing readers into their lives indicates their desires to live beyond the heartbreaking experience of losing a loved one. Recognizing that there is nothing they could have done to prevent the events is a way of acknowledging a desire to heal. By writing their stories, they express their willingness to keep Rising Stronger™.

I am in no way a grief expert. However, like our contributors and readers, my knowledge of the topic is pragmatic due to the loss of my grandparents, father, brother, best friend, and other close relatives and friends. Over the years, I faced near-death experiences with my two children. I experienced one child being read his last rights three times in one week, thinking it was the end. I am grateful that he overcame that obstacle. I held my seven-month-old child in my arms while he gasped for breath in a hospital in Kingston, Jamaica. He was immediately placed in an oxygen tent to save his life. If you have ever been in a situation where your children are making poor choices, you may understand my obsession with grief. If you are a terrified parent of losing a child, perhaps the real events in this book can also explain the importance of seeking help before it is too late.

Thank you for your continued support!
Keep Rising Stronger™!

For speaking engagement inquiries for the author and contributors, please contact me directly at

pwallner@nmwbglobal.com
www.nmwbglobal.com
www.paulinewallnerspeaks.com

For NMWB Global Management Services, LLC
Business Related Queries Only
Tel: 1-404-218-9176

Printed in the United States of America: Second Publication in the Rising Stronger Series™
Paperback: ISBN: 9781660076475